The Complete Idiot's Reference Card

A Quick Review of Common Cosmetic Procedures

Surgery: Face-Lift.
Cost: $7,500–$10,000.
Recovery time: Fast healers do well enough in 12 days. It is best to allow a full two weeks. If you are keeping a secret, allow four to six weeks. If you are taking pictures, in a wedding or such, allow three months, just to be safe.
Results: Face-lifts in healthy people last about 12 years. People who are fussy about their appearance might want maintenance as early as five years. If you are older, you might need maintenance sooner. If you do not take hormonal replacement, your face-lift will not last as long.

Surgery: Forehead Lift.
Cost: $5,000.
Recovery time: Fast healers who are only having their forehead done may be able to conceal the signs and be back to work in less than two weeks. If you bruise easily, the bruises can be covered with makeup and should not necessarily slow you down.
Results: Surgery for lines sometimes last as little as two to three years, but the elevation of the hairline is permanent. The loss of hair limits your ability to redo this surgery.

Surgery: Eyelids.
Cost: $4,500–$5,000 for surgery on both upper and lower lids, a bit more for Asian to Eurasian conversions.
Recovery time: Two to three weeks. You can get by with makeup under glasses or dark glasses.
Results: Can be very long lasting. They are usually done twice in a lifetime. Sometimes they can be refreshed (without open surgery) by a chemical peel.

Surgery: Nose.
Cost: $5,000–$10,000.
Recovery time: Cast is on for about 12 days. (The nose looks acceptable but swollen at the time.) This goes down substantially in the first three months, though there are swollen days during the first year. No glasses for the first three months; no sun or sleeping on your side for the same time.
Results: Can be permanent.

Surgery: Cheek Implants.
Cost: $4,500–$5,000.

Recovery: [...] bout after two [...] at its full [...] eople.
Results: Can be permanent.

Surgery: Chin Implant.
Cost: $3,500–$4,500.
Recovery time: For the first week after surgery you'll be on a liquid diet. You can be out and about soon after that, though you'll be somewhat swollen. The swelling should go down within three weeks.
Results: Can be permanent.

Surgery: Lip Fat Transplant.
Cost: $2,500, if under general anesthesia.
Recovery time: Two to three weeks.
Results: Results vary. Most successful for rejuvenating lips that have lost some of their fullness due to aging. Both younger patients and rejuvenation patients may require a second transplant after a year or two.

Procedure: Lip Collagen Injections.
Cost: $500.
Recovery time: Less than an hour.
Results: Can be very good and last two to three months, occasionally longer in certain patients.

Surgery: Neck Liposuction.
Cost: $4,200 with general anesthesia.
Recovery time: One week in bandages; however, some swelling persists into the second week in some people.
Results: Can be permanent. This procedure seems to protect against the need for a neck lift.

Surgery: Breast Augmentation.
Cost: $5,500–$7,200.
Recovery time: No driving for six days; no exercise or lifting for a month. It is recommended that you sleep alone the first two to three weeks. You can go back to work in a week or less.
Results: It is thought that a saline implant should last at least 10 years, though some have lasted as long as 30 years. Gel implants should be watched and likely changed when they are about 20 years old. The average young woman having breast surgery, because of maintenance and size changes, will have three surgeries in a lifetime.

ALPHA

Surgery: Breast Reduction.

Cost: $8,000–$8,500 for women; $5,000 for men.

Recovery time: You can return to work in five days. Bandages are necessary for three to four weeks. You should sleep alone for two to three weeks.

Results: Can be long-term but are not permanent. Touch-ups need not be complicated, and can include implants later in life.

Surgery: Pectoral Implants.

Cost: $7,200.

Recovery time: You are very tender for the first seven to ten days. Allow three weeks to recover.

Results: Can be long-term.

Surgery: Midsection Liposuction.

Cost: $6,000–$8,000, depending on size.

Recovery time: You are tender for about a week. You can go back to work in loose clothing after a week, but two to three weeks recovery is desirable.

Results: Can be permanent if you are weight stable and follow a good diet. It will not be successful if you have significant weight gain.

Surgery: Fanny Liposuction.

Cost: $5,000–$6,000.

Recovery time: About 10 days. You need two to three weeks to recover so that you can sit comfortably.

Results: Can be long-term, but you may need touching up.

Surgery: Thigh Liposuction.

Cost: $6,000–$8,000 for the entire thigh from below knee to hip, depending on size.

Recovery time: You are tender the first week but really need two weeks before going back to work, driving, and so on. You will need to wear an elastic stocking for three months after the surgery.

Results: Can be permanent even if weight is not stable.

Surgery: Arm Liposuction.

Cost: $5,000–$6,000, depending on size.

Recovery time: You can be out and about in a couple of days, but can't show your arms for about three weeks. You need to wear an elastic, long-sleeved shirt for two to three months.

Results: Can be long-term, if not permanent. The best results are in people who watch their diet and are healthy.

Surgery: Penis Enlargement.

Cost: Varies widely depending upon procedure.

Recovery time: Prolonged healing can vary between a few weeks to several months.

Results: Results are permanent. This surgery can result in deformity, erectile dysfunction, sexual dysfunction, and/or a decrease in sexual satisfaction. It is not recommended.

Surgery: Scar Revision.

Cost: Varies from $500–$5,000, depending on the degree of problem and the total length of the scars.

Recovery time: The wounds need to be splinted and made immobile for three weeks to get an optimal result. Sometimes not all the work should be done at one time. Scars that are too close to each other should not necessarily be fixed at the same time.

Results: Can achieve marked improvement. Generally scar revisions are worthwhile for the patient, though in unfavorable areas or on people with problem skin, the scars can become worse.

Surgery: Chemical Facial Peel.

Cost: $3,500–$4,000 for a medium-strength peel.

Recovery time: You should have fresh new skin in less than a week. This skin is dry and resistant to makeup for several days. The redness is well hidden under makeup over the next two months in the average person. Some people might stay red longer. Those who don't want the "bad sunburn" look can avoid attracting attention with applications of a minimal concealer.

Results: Can last as long as 15 years. Most results are very long-term and improve old face-lifts as well as prevent the need for other surgery later.

Surgery: Hair Transplants.

Cost: $5–$10 per graft.

Recovery time: About a week or less of dressings. You can be back to work with a hat or baseball cap in a day or two.

Results: Can be permanent. The transplanted hair will remain in place even if you continue to lose your original hair, which can produce unsatisfactory results.

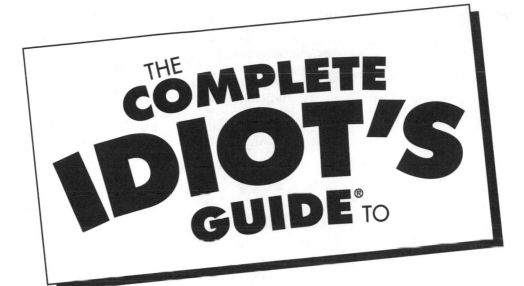

THE COMPLETE IDIOT'S GUIDE® TO

Cosmetic Surgery

by George Semel, M.D.
and Jeff St. John, Ph.D.

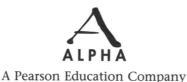

ALPHA

A Pearson Education Company

International Standard Book Number: 0-02-863993-6
Library of Congress Catalog Card Number: 2001088749

03 02 01   8 7 6 5 4 3 2 1

Interpretation of the printing code: The rightmost number of the first series of numbers is the year of the book's printing; the rightmost number of the second series of numbers is the number of the book's printing. For example, a printing code of 01-1 shows that the first printing occurred in 2001.

Printed in the United States of America

Publisher
Marie Butler-Knight

Product Manager
Phil Kitchel

Managing Editor
Jennifer Chisholm

Acquisitions Editor
Mike Sanders

Development Editor
Jennifer Moore

Production Editor
Billy Fields

Copy Editor
Amy Borrelli

Illustrator
Brian Moyer

Cover Designers
Mike Freeland
Kevin Spear

Book Designers
Scott Cook and Amy Adams of DesignLab

Indexer
Lisa Wilson

Layout/Proofreading
Mary Hunt
Natashia Rardin
Gloria Schurick

Contents at a Glance

Contents

Part 2: Heavenly Heads and Necks 57

5 Turning Heads and Breaking Hearts: Face-Lifts 59

6 Smoothing Out Your Forehead 69

Part 6: Happier Skin and Hair

23 Now You See It, Now You Don't: Scar Revision

Foreword

I have had the great pleasure of working with many legendary celebrities over the past 35 years as a make-up artist in Hollywood. Dr. George Semel is also a celebrity in his field. His renowned and respected research and work in reconstructive and plastic surgery have led to many innovations and advances in his field. Dr. Semel is more than a surgeon, he is a chemist and an artist. For more than twenty years of our professional association, his work and his profound vision have served as an inspiration to me and to the many thousands of make-up artists who have graduated from my schools and whom have received his fine tutelage.

When we first met, my many colleagues and I were introduced to the world of plastic surgery in a manner that enabled us as artists to rely upon him and to entrust the beauty of our clients to his skillful and artistic mind and hands. Throughout the years, I have had the pleasure to observe Dr. Semel's ability to understand every situation brought to him and to always be willing to unconditionally give his advice and assistance. Dr. Semel's passion for creating perfection through surgery has now evolved into the realm of skincare, thus making his genius available to everyone.

This book is a culmination of many years of care and dedication to all people who have known him. The uniqueness of this book is certainly a tribute to the outstanding knowledge that Dr. Semel has amassed throughout his brilliant career. The information which you are about to receive will provide you with a most complete and easy-to-understand explanation of every aspect of cosmetic surgery and scientifically produced skincare products and treatments. It is not often that information of this nature can be presented with such style and clarity. You may rest assured that the knowledge you are about to obtain is valid and has been supported by many years of professional inspiration. This book will most definitely provide you with the detailed knowledge and guidance necessary to understand every aspect of the procedures that you may be considering for yourself. I have entrusted many of my motion picture and television stars to Dr. Semel's care and, having read through this book, I know that you will not only enjoy it, but will understand why I, my graduates, and the majority of my colleagues have insisted that Dr. Semel be the real magician behind our make-up work.

Joe Blasco,

President & CEO,

Joe Blasco Make-up Centers

and Joe Blasco Cosmetics

Introduction

Cosmetic surgery can be a daunting process. No matter how old you are or how minor of an improvement you would like to make, surgery (or any other kind of cosmetic improvement) can be a confusing and scary proposition. This is why we have chosen to create a book that describes the who, what, when, where, why, and how much of cosmetic surgery and makes the entire process one that is simple and easy to understand. After reading this book, we believe that you will walk away with a clear understanding of when you need a good surgeon, when you need a good shrink, and what to expect before, during, and after any kind of cosmetic operation or procedure.

While we have tried to offer you the most up-to-date and useful information, this book does not express or imply guarantee or warranty of any kind. We encourage you to discuss the risks involved with any cosmetic procedure with your cosmetic surgeon.

How This Book Is Organized

We've organized this book to make it easy for you to find out how to improve upon a particular part of your body. We recommend that you read Part 1, "All You Need to Know to Plan a Successful Surgery" first, and then skip ahead to the part of the book that discusses the techniques you are most interested in learning about.

Part 1, "All You Need to Know to Plan a Successful Surgery," gives you the information you need to know before you ever step into a cosmetic surgeon's office for an initial consult. We tell you how you can determine if you're right for cosmetic surgery and whether cosmetic surgery is right for you. We also offer important advice about choosing a qualified cosmetic surgeon and discuss alternatives to surgery that you might want to consider before going under the knife.

Part 2, "Heavenly Heads and Necks," covers the cosmetic improvements available for your face and neck, including cosmetic dentistry, face- and neck-lifts, chemical peels and laser resurfacing, nose jobs, and lip enhancements. There are a surprising number of surgical and non-surgical things you can do to improve the appearance of your face and neck, and we cover them all in this part of the book.

Part 3, "Better Breasts and Chests," goes over the options available for improving the shape and/or size of your chest—whether you're a man or a woman. We discuss breast implants and lifts for women who want bigger or shapelier breasts and pectoral implants for guys who want more chest definition without working out.

Part 4, "Awesome Abdomens and Buttocks," looks at the ways you can improve the shape and size of your midsection and rear end. Many of the procedures available involve the use of liposuction, and we cover the basics of liposuction procedures in this part of the book.

Part 5, "Extremities and Other Things," examines the procedures that can be performed on the arms, thighs, calves, and penis to improve their appearance and make you feel better about yourself.

Part 6, "Happier Skin and Hair," shows you surgical and non-surgical options for improving the appearance of wrinkly or aging skin and covers the ins and outs of hair transplants and excess hair removal.

Part 7, "Let the Healing Begin!" encourages you to recognize that proper healing and recovery begins with proper preparation. We offer tips and advice to help you be as comfortable as possible during your recovery period.

Extras

Throughout this book you'll find boxes that will help guide you through the ins and outs of cosmetic surgery. The tips are divided into four categories and are repesented by their own special icons:

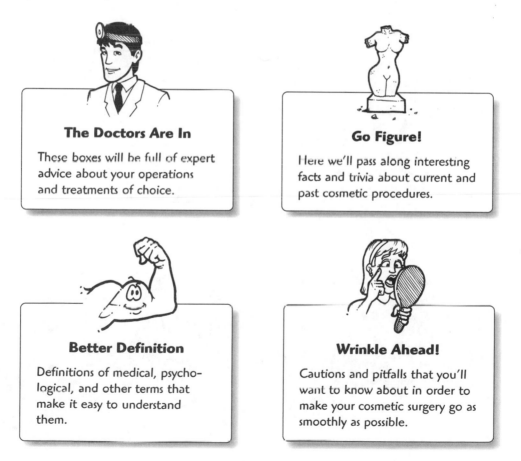

The Doctors Are In

These boxes will be full of expert advice about your operations and treatments of choice.

Go Figure!

Here we'll pass along interesting facts and trivia about current and past cosmetic procedures.

Better Definition

Definitions of medical, psychological, and other terms that make it easy to understand them.

Wrinkle Ahead!

Cautions and pitfalls that you'll want to know about in order to make your cosmetic surgery go as smoothly as possible.

Acknowledgments

We would like to extend a special note of thanks to the doctors and other professionals who have made this book possible. Our deepest gratitude goes out to Dr. Garry Corgiat, Dr. Greg Mueller, Dr. Michael Delmont, Dr. Derek Jones, Dr. Adrian Aiache, Dr. Harvy Abrams, Dr. William Rassman, Dr. Jean Kalle-Santikean, and Dr. Kate Bergam. In addition, it has been a pleasure for us to work with such great talents as Mike Sanders, Jennifer Moore, and the entire staff at Alpha Books. Your unwavering guidance and support throughout this entire project has been outstanding.

Trademarks

Part 1

All You Need to Know to Plan a Successful Surgery

An ancient proverb states that "the journey of a thousand miles begins with a single step," and this truth applies to cosmetic surgery. The first step to cosmetically improving your appearance is to define and learn the difference between beauty and cosmetic improvement, and to decide if either of these outcomes is what you hope to achieve. Gaining a clear understanding of the difference between these two goals is the only way that you will ever be able to estimate the outcome of your operation or be happy with any surgical result.

In order to alter your features, enhance physical characteristics, sculpt your figure or physique, or change your overall appearance, you'll also need to learn exactly what cosmetic surgery can and cannot accomplish for you. It is important to know its capabilities and its limitations and to know exactly how to get the best results that are available today. You'll need an action plan that is easy to understand, simple to follow, and realistic to maintain with your busy schedule.

With an abundance of new surgeries and procedures available today, it can be difficult to know which surgery or procedure is right for you. Learning where to begin, how to proceed, and what decision is right for you can often be overwhelming tasks.

As you will see, we've taken the confusion and frustration out of the cosmetic surgery process for you so that in the end, you can make a fully informed decision and feel completely comfortable and confident with your surgery of choice.

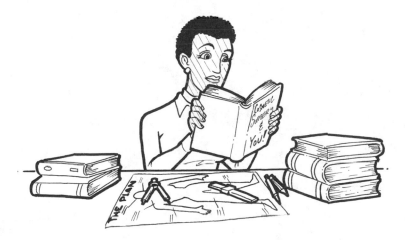

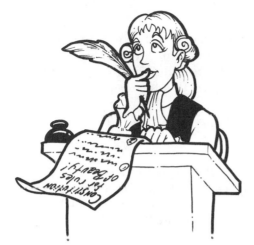

Chapter 1

Beauty Rules!

In This Chapter

➤ Defining beauty

➤ Finding out about what's out and what's in

➤ The psychology of cosmetic surgery

➤ Preparing mentally, emotionally, and financially for a successful surgery

There are as many definitions of beauty as there are beautiful people. Some people say beauty is only skin-deep, and that its definition is limited to an ideal collection of certain shapes and sizes of physical features. They believe that beauty is solely a physical trait and measured by how close someone's features fit particular aesthetic ideals. Others say that beauty is an inner quality that belongs to yet another select group of people. They believe that beauty is measured not by outward appearances but by the degree that someone recognizes his or her own self-worth, how well someone maintains an awareness of his or her own talents or abilities, and how well someone establishes a sense of confidence or self-esteem. They believe that beauty belongs only to those who have achieved these accomplishments.

What is an accurate definition of beauty that can help each of us to recognize our own inner and outer traits without excluding one or the other? We believe there is an easy answer to this question!

Defining Beauty

We believe that beauty does not belong to any select group of people. In fact, we know that everyone is beautiful. Every single person, no matter what age, weight, height, size, shape, race, and gender, is 100 percent beautiful—without exception. However, not everyone knows or chooses to recognize that he or she already possesses this quality.

Beauty Is a State of Being

Beauty is a condition that each of us is born into that develops as a result of the maturation of our own self-awareness and physical features. Owning your own beauty begins with a basic understanding that you are indeed a beautiful human being, regardless of whether or not your outward appearance fits society's ever-changing definitions of beauty. Without this basic knowledge, no amount of surgery will ever be able to change your mind, and you will want to cosmetically alter your appearance whenever a new fad appears on the fashion scene.

Own Your Beauty

If you own your own beauty, it will be reflected in your outward appearance and make you more attractive to others. When you believe you are already beautiful, you will feel beautiful. When you feel beautiful, your mood will most likely be more attractive to others because your expressions and gestures will be free from insecurity and self-doubt. Others will probably be attracted to your personality and can appreciate your facial features better when they are not wrinkled from worry or scrunched up by self-doubt. They can more easily see the beautiful color of your eyes when they are not looking downward or away out of self-consciousness, and they can more easily notice your radiant smile when it is not covered by the frown that you wear when you are feeling unattractive.

Being beautiful begins by believing that you are already beautiful. This belief can change your entire appearance all by itself! We suggest that you make this your very first cosmetic improvement, if you haven't done so already.

Look at Yourself in a New Light

Before you seek cosmetic improvements to your appearance, we recommend that you look at any physical features that you consider to be unattractive in a completely different light. Try to look at your physical imperfections as "special imperfections." View them as physical traits that make you unique and set you apart from all the rest. Be proud of the distinct features that you possess. Just because a physical feature is unusual, doesn't necessarily mean that it has to be considered unattractive. Others will tend to respond to your appearance the same way that you respond to your appearance—if you like it, they'll tend to like it.

Set Your Own Beauty Standards

We recommend that you set your own standard of personal beauty. We suggest that you decide for yourself what physical features you can live with and what ones you would rather live without. We encourage you to determine what size and shape you want your physical features to be and never to lose sight of the fact that you are already a beautiful person.

When you set your own personal standard of physical beauty, you will probably be less likely to be persuaded by others to alter your appearance. Any cosmetic improvements that are made to your appearance should be self-motivated and not at the request or insistence of those you know. We also encourage you to remember that what is in style and considered to be attractive today, may not be considered attractive years from now when fashion changes. So, be sure that you will be satisfied with your cosmetic results—and will be satisfied years down the road.

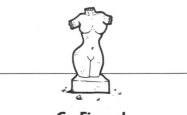

Go Figure!

There are plenty of people who have taken what might be considered a physical imperfection and made it their beauty trademark. Supermodel Cindy Crawford has never had her facial mole removed. In fact, it has become a trait that she is famous for, and she is world-renowned for setting the standard for beauty in the fashion industry. If she can live with a facial mole, what physical feature can you live with as a "perfect imperfection"?

International Standards of Beauty

If you already believe that you are a beautiful person and you have chosen what physical features you can live with as perfect imperfections, you may still decide that there are some cosmetic improvements that you would like to have made. You might want to take a look at what international beauty experts currently consider to be "beautiful" features. Keep in mind that these standards usually change over time and are only meant to give you some ideas to make up your own mind about how you would like to cosmetically improve your appearance.

Physical features have been agreed upon in international circles for quite a while. Cosmetic surgeons around the world have found that those seeking cosmetic surgery have similar goals in mind when it comes to improving their appearances. The most popular requested improvements to facial features are listed here.

A Fair Complexion

A fair complexion that is blemish-free, even in color and tone, and smooth in texture is a popular cosmetic improvement that many people seek. People of all color frequently request that their complexion be lightened for a more vibrant complexion. This usually reduces or eliminates the appearances of blemishes, scars, and uneven skin tone.

A Narrow Nose with the Tip of the Nose as the Highest Part (sticking out farther than the chin, cheek, or forehead)

Noses that have a tip that is lower than the rest of the nose or nostrils that are naturally wide are frequently seen as problematic for those who seek cosmetic improvement. Most patients and surgeons agree that the tip of the nose should be the highest part of the nose that stands away from the face and that nostrils should be narrow. Bumps that were frequently removed in the past are often left in place but minimized in order to give the nose a more natural appearance.

Noticeable Cheekbones

Cheekbones are often not formed from bone but from fat deposits that are present in youth and absorbed with age. It causes the appearance of cheekbones to disappear over time. These can be replaced with cheek implants to make your cheekbones as noticeable as they were when you were younger.

A Strong Chin

Many people who have what surgeons call "weak chins" or chins that are not slightly pronounced or defined are common candidates for chin implants. Chin implants can give the appearance of a strong chin. Chins are a part of what determines facial shape and can be used to alter the contour of your face.

Well-Defined Eyes

Eyes that are well defined and free of extra skin, heavy lids, or unwanted bags underneath are commonly requested. Also, lids that have lost a lot of fat due to age are common candidates for fat transplants to fill the emptied skin that sags without the natural fat and tissue to fill it. Both conditions can be cosmetically improved.

Full Lips

Lips that are full and natural in appearance are a popular request. Everyone seems to want fuller-shaped lips without looking like they just stepped out of the operating room. This is possible with today's techniques.

Symmetrical Features

Everyone's body is naturally asymmetrical—meaning that one side of the body is a little different in shape and size than the other. However, most people agree that they would like their features, particularly their eyes, ears, and breasts, to be as close to the exact same shape and size as possible. Symmetrical features are highly desired—but almost a surgical impossibility. However, some improvement can be made.

These are some ideas that can help you decide how you might want to have your facial features cosmetically improved. There might be other parts of your body that you would like to have surgically altered, too. If this is the case, check out the other exciting chapters in this book for the surgeries and procedures that apply to your cosmetic needs!

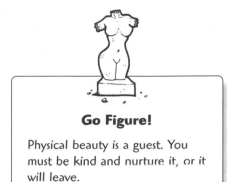

Go Figure!

Physical beauty is a guest. You must be kind and nurture it, or it will leave.

The Psychology of Cosmetic Surgery

When you approach cosmetic surgery with the mind-set that you are already a beautiful person and you just want to make a few cosmetic improvements to your appearance, you increase your chances of being satisfied with your surgery. You are not relying on surgery to make you beautiful; instead, you are relying on it to make a slight improvement to a physical feature or features.

The Right Beauty Mind-Set

Once your surgery is complete, you will undoubtedly evaluate whether or not it was a success, and you'll determine whether or not you like your results. Your evaluation of your results will be very different depending on your mind-set at the time!

➤ If your mind-set after your surgery is that the surgery itself is completely responsible for making you feel and look beautiful, then you will judge the success of your surgery based on how you feel about yourself (your self-esteem) after your surgery, rather than how you feel about the physical results of your operation. The two are completely different and the success of your surgery should be based on the physical results rather that a fluctuating sense of self-esteem.

➤ If you come in with the mind-set that you are already beautiful, you will judge the success of your surgery based on the actual cosmetic improvements that were surgically made to one or more of your physical features. You will be able to assess the success of your surgery more accurately and with more realistic expectations.

Keep in mind, surgery alone cannot give you a solid sense of beauty if you did not walk into the operating room with at least a little bit of it already built in! It can only enhance what is already there.

How You Feel Going in Determines How You'll Feel Coming Out

Studies have shown that patients who did not have a solid sense of their own beauty when they walked into surgery came out being very unhappy with their results, regardless of how well the results looked to everyone else after the operation. These patients tended not to see themselves as the same person with an improved physical feature; instead, they tended to see themselves as the same person with the same unaltered feature. They still saw themselves with the same physical imperfection after their surgery as they did before their surgery due to low self-esteem and a distorted body image. This is why it is so important to have a strong sense of your own beauty before your surgery and not to look towards cosmetic surgery as a cure-all for feelings of physical deficits. (Maxwell Maltz also found that people who had a sense of their own beauty had an increased sense of beauty after a successful cosmetic surgery was performed!)

Cosmetic surgery is not for those with severe self-esteem issues or for those who cannot accurately perceive their own body image (see Chapter 2, "Are You Right for Cosmetic Surgery?"). Be sure that you have the proper mind-set before you consider making any kind of cosmetic improvement to your appearance. As Dr. Garry Corgiat, a noted psychologist and celebrity of the TV show "Shrink Talk" puts it, "A surgical solution can never be a remedy for any psychological problem."

Beauty Marks

Cosmetic surgeries of the past have left what we call "beauty marks." Beauty marks are the telltale signs of fads and fashions that have left the cosmetic scene just as quickly as they became a permanent part of some people's bodies through surgery or some kind of cosmetic procedure. They are the hair transplants that left the "plugged" look in men during the 1970s and the silicone-injected lips that migrated to other parts of some women's bodies during the early 1980s. These are just a few examples!

Unfortunately, these beauty marks come much easier than they go. They are a permanent part of many people's appearances, unless they had their appearance altered back to their original state, if it was surgically possible. Here is a list of old techniques and procedures that left telltale signs of surgery or "beauty marks," versus the new techniques and procedures that create a more natural-looking appearance. Be aware of past and present techniques!

What's Out	What's In
Injections of silicone	Injections of fat
Overcorrected Asian eyes	Natural double lid
Undercorrected Asian eyes	Natural double lid
Hollow eyes that are round	Oval eyes that are elongated
Cheekbones that are too big	Subtle improvement of cheekbones
Lips that are too big	Restoration of curve and fullness to lips
Tweezed pencil-line eyebrows	Normal-shaped brows
Noses that are too small	Natural, refined noses
Chins that are too big	Subtle improvement of form
High foreheads	Normal-height foreheads, but smooth
High eyebrows	Eyebrows at level they were in high school
Bright makeup tattoo	Permanent makeup, if any, is subtle
Early surgical overcorrection	Fat transplants to restore youthful fat and contours
Laser resurfacing	Chemical peels and occasional light dermabrasion
Hair transplants	Follicular-unit transplants
Laser for veins	Injections for veins

Review this list before you decide to visit your local cosmetic surgeon. Becoming aware of the most up-to-date procedures for cosmetic improvement can save you time, money, and, most of all, your beautiful appearance! In addition, it will also be helpful for you to know if you are a candidate for any kind of cosmetic surgery or procedure.

Beauty Procedures and Age

Below is a list of the most common surgeries and procedures that are currently performed by many surgeons, and the minimum age requirements for candidacy. More information on these surgeries and their candidacy are listed throughout the other chapters of this book.

➤ **Face-lifts:** Most people are not candidates for this surgery until 40 years of age and over.

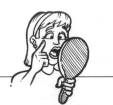

Wrinkle Ahead!

Telltale signs of cosmetic surgery are a risk with any cosmetic procedure, and you need to make sure that you fully understand the possible problems and are fully prepared for the possibility that they could happen to you. Cosmetic surgery is never completely risk free!

➤ **Forehead:** Candidates for this surgery are over 18 or have finished growing. The most ideal candidates have low foreheads and thick, dark, hair.

➤ **Eyes:** Most candidates for eye surgery are over 40, but anyone over 18 can qualify if congenital fat is considered to be problematic or if a change of feature shape is desired.

➤ **Nose:** Anyone over the age of 18 who is finished growing can be a candidate for this surgery. We suggest that candidates wait until they are finished growing so that they and their surgeons can adequately assess what size and shape of nose would go well with their adult features.

➤ **Lips:** Anyone over 18 is a candidate for this surgery unless there is a birth defect or physical abnormality present. In this case, any age is acceptable, provided that the child initially expresses a desire for surgery.

➤ **Ears:** Ear surgery is one of the most common cosmetic procedures that are performed on children. This surgery can be performed on anyone over five years old. However, the child must want to have the surgery performed and express to his or her parents that he or she would like to be considered for the operation. This is not a surgery for parents to insist that their children have performed.

➤ **Neck:** Most people are not candidates for cosmetic improvements (neck-lifts) to be made to their necks until they are age 40 and above. Some people qualify as candidates for neck liposuction if they are genetically predisposed to have fatty necks. In this case, the minimum age for neck liposuction is 18 years of age.

➤ **Cosmetic dentistry:** After a full set of adult teeth have developed, anyone can be considered to be a candidate for cosmetic dentistry.

➤ **Breast augmentation:** This is a surgery that we highly recommend women wait until they are well into their adulthood to consider. This is not the type of surgery to enter into without lengthy evaluation. For those young people who insist on having this surgery performed, the minimum age requirement for breast augmentation is 18—it's the law in some states!

➤ **Breast reduction:** The minimum age we recommend for this surgery is 18. However, we strongly suggest that women wait until they are well into adulthood to make such an important decision that will severely alter their appearance. However, some young women are candidates for liposuction techniques that leave minimal scars. We also recommend that women wait until their bodies stop developing to have the surgery performed so that more surgery is not required later.

➤ **Pectorals:** Pectoral implants for men are considered to be an option for men over the age of 21.

➤ **Tummies:** Tummy tucks are not recommended unless you are over 40 and have extreme amounts of excess skin due to severe weight fluctuation or skin that has completely lost its elasticity due to age, hormonal loss, or sun damage.

➤ **Liposuction in your mid-section:** Anyone over 18 qualifies as a candidate for this surgery. However, we strongly urge young people to practice a healthy diet and active lifestyle before seeking liposuction as a tummy-trimming option. Most young people tend to have metabolisms that respond more quickly to diet and exercise and cause more rapid weight loss. They also have skin that con-tracts more easily than the skin of older adults.

➤ **Fannies:** Fanny tucks are usually reserved for those over 40 who have extreme amounts of excess skin due to severe weight fluctuation and loss of skin elastic-ity. Liposuction is commonly performed on the fannies of other people and the age of candidacy for this procedure is over 18. However, we only recommend that this surgery be performed on older adults.

➤ **Thighs (lifts and liposuction):** Traditional thigh lifts of the past are rarely used today and are frequently reserved for those over the age of 40 whose legs have lost their shape due to severe weight fluctuation and loss of skin elasticity. Liposuction of the thighs can be performed as early as age 18.

➤ **Arms:** Traditional arm lifts of the past are also commonly reserved for those over 40 who have extreme amounts of excess skin due to weight loss. Liposuction of the arms is also usually reserved for women over 40 but can be performed on patients as young as 18.

➤ **Calves:** Candidates for calf-implantation surgery are age 18 and over. We highly recommend that people of all ages attempt to gain the shape and size of calves that they want through exercise first. Professional bodybuilders need not apply for this surgery because it will disqualify them for most major competitions.

➤ **Penis enlargement:** We recommend that no one apply for the lengthening and girth-producing surgeries that are available today. Our chapter on penis enlarge-ments in this book does offer some other interesting alternatives. Candidacy for these techniques begin at age 21 unless there is a birth defect or trauma that needs reconstructive surgery.

➤ **Facial skin:** Candidacy for soft-tissue-augmentation procedures begin at age 18. However, it is usually reserved only for those over the age of at least 30.

➤ **Hair transplants:** Most people commonly become candidates for this surgery in their 30s and 40s. Those who suffer from hair loss earlier than that can also be considered candidates. The minimum age requirement that we recommend for this surgery is 18. Remember to try to prevent hair loss with drug intervention.

➤ **Hair removal:** Anyone over the age of 18 is a candidate for this cosmetic procedure. Anyone younger than age 18 must have written parental permission in order to have laser hair removal performed. The earlier it is treated, the better.

We hope these age requirements have helped you to determine whether or not you may be a candidate for some of these cosmetic procedures and surgeries. Check out the other chapters of this book to discover more interesting facts about the surgeries and details about candidacy.

Beauty Rules!

Everyone wants to improve his or her physical appearance in the quickest and easiest way possible. We realize this and want to help you achieve your cosmetic goals. In order to fulfill your cosmetic improvement wish list, we've put together some of the most common beauty rules to help make your treatment of choice a success. Here are some tidbits of conventional wisdom that those "in the know" put into practice when they are considering any kind of cosmetic surgery.

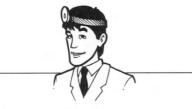

The Doctors Are In

You have the right to make a fully informed decision! Make sure your doctor answers all of your questions. If he or she doesn't supply the information you request, then find a different doctor!

Rules for Physical Preparation

Cosmetic surgeries are entirely elective procedures that you can have a great amount of control over. You have the responsibility to make sure that you fully understand the procedure you choose, but you also have the right to demand the highest quality treatment available. Follow these rules to ensure a successful surgery:

You have the right to make an informed decision.

You have a right to know everything about your surgery, from the professional history of your surgeon, to how the surgery will be performed, to how much the surgery will cost. Don't be afraid to ask questions. This is your surgery and you have the right to know as much about your operation as possible before you schedule a surgery date.

You have the right to confidential treatment.

Your medical history and any current treatment you are receiving should be completely confidential. Your doctor does not have the legal right to discuss your treatment with other people or the treatment of other patients with you unless a *release form* or *consent form* has been signed.

If your surgeon discusses your treatment with others without your written permission or discusses someone else's treatment with you without signed consent, he or she is breaking the law.

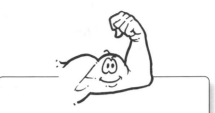

Better Definition

A **release form** or **consent form** states exactly to whom the doctor has permission to disclose the details of the patient's treatment.

You have the right to get the results that you want.

Make sure that the surgeon you choose to perform your operation fully understands and is capable of making the cosmetic improvements that you want made. Avoid selecting a doctor who has his or her mind set on giving you a certain result if it is not one that you are absolutely certain that you would like.

Do not choose a surgeon who insists on giving all of his or her patients the same look (such as the same shape eyes, the same shape nose, the same size cheekbones, etc.). You probably will not want to look exactly like every other patient that this doctor has ever operated on. Remember, it is your surgery and you will have to live with the results!

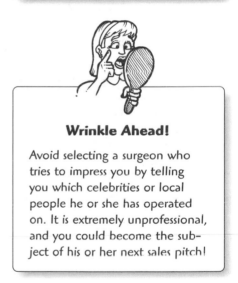

Wrinkle Ahead!

Avoid selecting a surgeon who tries to impress you by telling you which celebrities or local people he or she has operated on. It is extremely unprofessional, and you could become the subject of his or her next sales pitch!

You have the right to stop at any time.

Some people feel obligated to follow through with having a cosmetic surgery performed, even after they have decided that surgery would not be in their best interest. All too often, they feel guilty about canceling their cosmetic surgery plans after an initial consultation because they are afraid of disappointing their surgeon or feel obliged to pay his or her full surgical fee when surgery has not been performed. In this case, they are actually only responsible for the services that have been rendered to date (that is, the fee for initial consultation).

You can stop your cosmetic surgery plans at any time before your surgery; you are not obligated to follow through if you suddenly have a change of heart. The only time it is not advisable for you to stop treatment is during or after your surgery, when complications arise that pose physical danger or significant distress (like infection, bleeding, or abnormal healing). You are not obligated to receive any future treatment other than follow-up exams to ensure proper healing which could take weeks or months.

Rules for Mental and Emotional Preparation

Whereas the actual results of your surgery are in a large part determined by the skill of the surgeon you choose, your emotional state after the surgery is in your hands. Make sure you are prepared for the surgery by following these guidelines:

Personalize your surgery.

You are the only person who will have to wear the results of your surgery. You are the primary person who will have to live with the face and the body that is wheeled out of the operating room. For this reason, we suggest that you personalize your surgery so that the results fit your unique tastes and desired appearance.

Don't be afraid to request something that other people might not want. For instance, say you've got a small bump on your nose and nostrils that are a little wide for your taste, and you've decided to have your nose done. However, the reason you want the operation is not to have the small bump removed, but only to narrow your nostrils just a little bit, because that is what will accurately suit your tastes. Other people who have the same surgery performed might insist on having their bump removed. Don't be afraid to personalize your surgery so that it fits your tastes and appearance of choice. You and you alone will be the one to wear the results!

Be sure that you are doing this for you.

Do not allow yourself to be talked into permanently altering your appearance by any-one for any reason. We strongly suggest that any and all cosmetic improvements you make be self-motivated in order for you to truly be pleased with your results. If you don't want the surgery to begin with, you certainly won't be happy with the results after your surgery is finished. Those who try to persuade others into having un-wanted or unnecessary surgery usually stand to gain something from the results themselves. Beware of agendas! Proceed with surgery only if it is what you want for yourself and not what somebody else wants for you!

Talk to someone who has already had the surgery.

Use the buddy system! Many people decide to have cosmetic surgery performed after they have noticed remarkable results that a friend received. We suggest that you choose a friend to talk to before and after your surgery so you'll have the support you'll need during this transitional time. Someone who has had cosmetic surgery or a surgery similar to the one that you'll have performed would be the ideal person for you to confide in, granted that he or she can keep a secret!

Decide if it is going to be a secret.

Most people prefer to keep their cosmetic surgery a secret. They would like for others to think that their appearance is one that Mother Nature gave them rather than one that their cosmetic surgeon created for them. They may only disclose their secret to their closest friends. We understand the reasons why most people choose not to disclose the fact that they've had surgery, and we encourage you to determine whether or not it matters to you if others know that you have had cosmetic surgery. If you do want to keep your surgery a secret, you'll want to pay close attention to the postoperative section of each chapter of this book so that you will know when you can resume your social activities and still keep your secret … a secret!

Determine your own rules about disclosure.

Different people have different rules about disclosure when it comes to cosmetic surgery. Some people don't want anyone to know, some people don't mind if their closest friends know, and others don't care if everybody knows! We suggest that you determine your own rules about disclosure. Here are two examples: Determine whom you can tell and why you can tell them about your surgery. You might decide you can only tell your family members because you know that they will keep your secret. Or, you might decide to tell your close group of friends about your surgery because you know that they will not judge you or think of you as vain for electing to have cosmetic surgery performed. Or, you might decide that you can tell everyone about your surgery because you want all of them to know which surgeon to go to when they need to have a similar surgery performed.

Don't make any hasty decisions.

Don't let eagerness get the best of you when you decide to have your surgery. Take your time to learn all the facts and risks about the operation you are considering. The surgery you are contemplating today will still be there tomorrow, unless it is replaced with a quicker and more effective treatment. In that case, you'll be even happier that you waited!

Be sure of your decision before you schedule surgery.

Avoid planning a surgery that you are really undecided about having. Many people make a down payment for a surgery that they are unsure about, thinking that this will give them greater motivation to have the surgery later on. In many cases like these, fear or better judgment frequently prevails and a significant amount of money is lost. Be sure of your decision before you schedule your surgery.

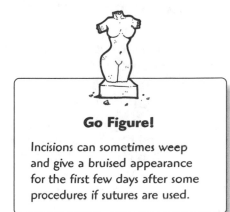

Go Figure!

Incisions can sometimes weep and give a bruised appearance for the first few days after some procedures if sutures are used.

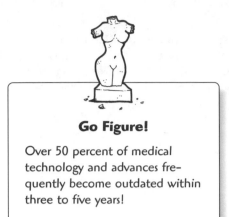

Go Figure!

Over 50 percent of medical technology and advances frequently become outdated within three to five years!

Take the next available appointment.

Many people worry about going in for surgery even after they have clearly decided that they want to have the surgery performed. If this is you, we recommend that you take the next appointment that your doctor has available. This will give you less time to worry and get you the results that you want more quickly.

Expect pain … and do it anyway!

We won't sugarcoat the truth by telling you that you might feel "some discomfort" after your surgery. The truth is that most surgeries cause some postoperative pain! You will experience some pain, even with painkillers, and you can anticipate this result no matter how well you plan your operation or your recovery period. If you've learned all the facts and risks about your surgery and you are certain that you still want to have the operation performed, expect to feel some pain … and do it anyway!

Stay busy up until the time of your surgery.

If you have taken the next available appointment that was offered to you, you still might have to wait at least a week or two before you can actually have your surgery performed. You will most likely need this time to prepare for your surgery by having blood tests performed and by eliminating certain ingredients from your blood system that can complicate your surgery (like aspirin). All of these will take time! While you are in the process of getting ready, try to schedule additional activities for yourself if you think that you might have too much free time on your hands that will be spent worrying about your surgery. Try to stay busy and keep your mind preoccupied right up until the time of your surgery!

Rules for Financial Preparation

Cosmetic surgery isn't cheap, and because it is an elective procedure intended for aesthetic reasons alone, it usually isn't covered by medical insurance. Read on to find out how to prepare for the financial aspects of your cosmetic procedure.

Save!

To make your surgery the least expensive and cost-effective as possible, we recommend that you save enough money to pay for your surgery in full (or as close to as full as possible) at the time of your operation.

Get at least three price quotes.

We recommend that you consult with at least three surgeons and obtain at least three price quotes to learn what the average price of your surgery is in your area. Prices can vary depending on location. Avoid reserving a surgery date with the first surgeon you meet until you talk with other doctors in your area and do some comparison-price shopping. This could save you hundreds and possibly even thousands of dollars!

Consider choosing a surgeon who charges an average price.

Consider choosing a surgeon who charges a price that is in the average range of cost for your operation. In some cases, this can give you the greatest amount of cosmetic improvement for the least amount of money. Many surgeons who charge the going rate for surgery have chosen their prices according to what they have discovered is a standard price to charge over the course of their career in medicine. They have been around long enough to know both the market and the demand for surgeries and what is a fair price to pay. The "going rate" can sometimes reflect longevity and credibility of practice.

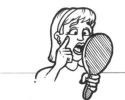

Wrinkle Ahead!

Many people who seek cosmetic surgery plan to pay for their operation or procedure by charging it on their credit card and paying the minimum balance due each month. This is an extremely expensive method of paying for your cosmetic improvement. You might end up paying hundreds and possibly even thousands of dollars in interest over the next few years while you pay for your surgery in monthly installments.

Be willing to spend more if the results will be better.

We recommend that one of your cosmetic goals be to get the absolute best cosmetic result that is available to you at a price that you can afford. If you have saved properly for your operation and funds are available, we suggest that you be willing to spend a little bit more money than the average cost of your surgery if the results will be better. Check out your doctor's postoperative results to get a good idea of what your money can afford you. You won't want to bargain with your appearance!

The most expensive is not always the best.

Just because a surgeon charges more for his or her services than all the other surgeons in the area does not mean that he or she can give you the best cosmetic results. Avoid believing the myth that the most expensive surgeon is always the best surgeon for you. Let a surgeon's history of successful results determine whom you choose to perform your surgery, not the price that he or she charges for your operation.

Beware of discount treatment.

Discount treatment is sometimes a promotional strategy that is used to increase sales of surgeries by new practices or places of business that have experienced a decrease in revenue. Most well-established surgeons usually do not need to offer such discounted treatments; other surgeons who respect their work tend to refer a large number of patients to them. Other well-established surgeons have performed enough successful surgeries that the word of mouth from their satisfied patients keeps their operating rooms full. The most common exception to this rule is that it is sometimes customary for a doctor to discount his or her services when they are offered to other doctors or those doctors' families.

Get an itemized list.

Remember, you are entitled to make a fully informed decision about your surgery, and that includes knowing in advance exactly what it is that you will be expected to pay. Ask your surgeon for an itemized list of costs for all the things your surgery will require. This way you will know exactly what to anticipate. You will also avoid paying for any hidden or additional costs by following this advice!

Plan for follow-up treatments.

Most surgeries require follow-up treatments in order to maintain the appearance of your cosmetic improvement. Implants are commonly replaced over the course of a person's lifetime, and lifts of any kind (especially face-lifts) might need to be redone every 12 years or so. Keep this in mind, and include follow-up treatments in your cosmetic surgery budget.

Expect the unexpected.

Occasionally, unforeseen complications do arise during and after surgery. No matter how well you and your surgeon plan your operation or recovery period, there is always a risk of complications (such as excessive bleeding, pulling a stitch, infection, lack of desirable healing or improper skin contraction, and so on). This might result in additional cost to you. Ask your doctor about his or her payment policies on treatment for unforeseen complications.

Get Ready for a Beautiful Journey!

These are the most common beauty rules that people who seek surgery safely practice before their operation or procedure. We recommend that you keep these rules in mind as you begin your journey of personal transformation.

Welcome to the wonderful world of cosmetic surgery, and good luck on completing your cosmetic surgery goals!

> **The Least You Need to Know**
>
> ➤ Know that you are already a beautiful person.
>
> ➤ Cosmetic surgery cannot make you beautiful; it can only improve the appearance of physical features.
>
> ➤ Save and try to pay the complete bill for your cosmetic surgery at the time of your operation.
>
> ➤ Make an informed decision.
>
> ➤ You have the right to confidential treatment.

Chapter 2

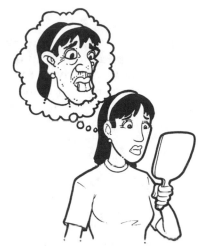

Are You Right for Cosmetic Surgery?

In This Chapter

➤ Determining whether you're turning to cosmetic surgery to improve your appearance or to try to improve your life in ways that no surgery will ever achieve

➤ Eating disorders and psychological problems that you should be aware of

➤ Honing in on problem areas of your body that cosmetic surgery can improve

➤ The difference between cosmetic surgery advocacy and addiction

You've decided you want a cosmetic procedure and you have enough money to pay for it ... so you're ready to schedule your operation, right? Wrong! Just because you have the desire and the funds to have a procedure performed, it doesn't necessarily mean that you are right for cosmetic surgery ... or that it is right for you.

There are many things you should consider before scheduling any kind of operation, and especially one that will permanently change your physical appearance. If you are unhappy with certain aspects of your personality or depressed about particular circumstances in your life, no amount of surgery will ever be able to correct these nonsurgical issues. This chapter will help you to understand when you are right for cosmetic surgery, and when cosmetic surgery is right for you!

When You Are Right for Cosmetic Surgery

Deciding that you are right for cosmetic surgery requires you to take an honest look at yourself—inside and out. Cosmetic surgery can fix how you appear to the rest of the world, but it can't fix the way that you see yourself if you don't already do so realistically. For instance, if you see yourself as a fat person when the rest of the world sees you as someone who is of average weight (or possibly even underweight), all of the liposuction in the world isn't going to change the way you see yourself. In this case the problem isn't your weight, but that you perceive yourself to be fat when in fact you are really not overweight at all. This is an example of what mental-health-care professionals call a distorted body image.

Many people suffer from a distorted body image and don't accurately see their bodies in the same way that the rest of the world does. Some even suffer from an acute case of a distorted body image called body dysmorphia, which will be explained later in this chapter. Having a distorted body image is a common problem today among many women, especially teens, and even among a growing number of men and adolescent boys.

Before you determine whether cosmetic surgery is right for you, you should rule out the possibility that your problem is psychological (like depression or a distorted body image) and needs to be treated with counseling or psychiatric medication. You'll want to make sure that you do not seek a surgical solution to a psychological problem. If you do, you will never be satisfied! It won't matter how beautiful or perfect everyone else thinks you look after you've healed from your surgery, you will still feel unhappy—no operation will be able to please you.

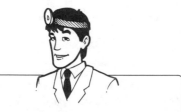

The Doctors Are In

The best candidates for cosmetic surgery are those who want to improve their outward appearance, not those who want to change their self-perception, self-esteem, or difficult situations in their lives that are unrelated to how they look.

If you are depressed about life's circumstances, a cosmetic procedure won't elevate your mood—just your skin! Remember, your surgeon will be operating with a knife, not a magic wand, and you'll be leaving his office with painkillers, not antidepressants. After you leave, you will be returning to your regularly scheduled life … and all of the circumstances that go with it.

When determining whether or not a psychological problem is your main motivation for surgery, ask yourself if you are generally happy and if you are satisfied with most or all aspects of your life. Do you like who you are, but dislike the way you look in the mirror? Or, do you dislike the person looking back at you—you!—and think that surgery will boost your self-esteem? Is your life already fulfilling, or are you expecting surgery to improve the quality of your life and not just your looks? These are important questions to ask yourself when deciding if you are right for cosmetic surgery.

Eating Disorders and Other Psychological Problems

You should also familiarize yourself with the signs and symptoms of common eating disorders and other treatable psychological problems that drive people into the operating rooms of cosmetic surgeons. If you have any of these problems, cosmetic surgery is not the answer!

The three most common eating disorders are *anorexia nervosa, bulimia nervosa,* and *binge-eating disorder.* Any of these eating disorders can strike anyone at anytime and commonly affect people who already suffer from some form of depression or anxiety, or those who already suffer from some degree of distorted body image (like body dysmorphia). If you meet any of the criteria for these conditions, cosmetic surgery won't be a solution.

Anorexia Nervosa

Someone affected by anorexia nervosa refuses to maintain a body weight at or above average for his or her height and age. According to the *Diagnostic and Statistical Manual* used by mental-health professionals, a person with anorexia nervosa weighs less than 85 percent of what would be considered the average for his or her height and age.

Anorexia nervosa is also characterized by an intense fear of gaining weight or becoming fat (even though the person is underweight), a distorted body image, denial of current low weight, and amenorrhea (the absence of at least three consecutive menstrual cycles in postmenarcheal women).

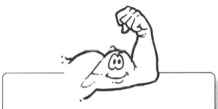

Better Definition

Anorexia Nervosa is an eating disorder characterized by self-starvation due to a distortion of body image.

Bulimia Nervosa

Bulimia nervosa involves recurrent episodes of binge eating and forms of purging. When someone suffers from bulimia nervosa, he or she eats an abnormally large amount of food in a short period of time that someone else of the same height, body frame, and age would not normally eat under similar circumstances. Also, he or she experiences a lack of self-control during binging (consuming large amounts of food) and feels like he or she cannot stop.

Other symptoms of bulimia nervosa include purging behaviors (such as the misuse of laxatives, diuretics, enemas, and other medications),

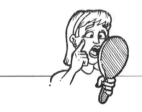

Wrinkle Ahead!

Males don't suffer from anorexia nervosa, right? Wrong! Anyone—male or female, adolescent or adult—can have anorexia nervosa, and doctors have been diagnosing many more men and boys with the problem than they did in the past.

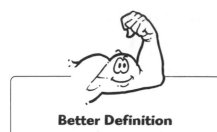

Better Definition

Bulimia Nervosa is an eating disorder characterized by cycles of bingeing (overeating) and self-induced purging (vomiting or overuse of laxatives).

self-induced vomiting, excessive exercise, or fasting to prevent weight gain. When someone exhibits these behaviors on an average of twice a week for a period of three months, he or she meets the criteria of someone suffering from bulimia nervosa.

Binge-Eating Disorder

Binge-eating disorder is characterized by recurrent episodes of binge eating. It is a similar condition to bulimia nervosa, except the purging behaviors are absent. If someone has a binge-eating disorder, he or she will eat an unusually large amount of food in a two-hour period of time that another person of the same height and age would not normally eat.

This common disorder frequently results in obesity and can lead to health problems such as heart attack, stroke, and diabetes. But you do not have to be overweight or at risk for any of these health problems to be diagnosed with a binge-eating disorder. People of all different shapes, sizes, and weights suffer from binge eating. When someone exhibits bingeing behaviors on an average of twice a week for three months, then he or she meets the criteria for binge-eating disorder.

Depression

Depression has many different indications, including a depressed mood, feelings of emptiness or irritability, reduced interest in pleasurable activities, significant weight loss or weight gain (more than 5 percent per month), insomnia (decrease in ability to sleep) or hypersomnia (chronic sleeping), sluggishness or fatigue, feelings of worthlessness, inappropriate guilt, reduced ability to concentrate, and suicidal thoughts or a preoccupation with death. Five or more of these features must be present for at least two weeks for someone to meet the criteria for being clinically depressed.

Body Dysmorphia

Body dysmorphia is a severe case of distorted body image. Someone suffering from body dysmorphia has an extreme preoccupation with a slight physical imperfection or imagined defect in his or her appearance. This imperfection causes the person such severe distress that it impairs his or her ability to function normally in social situations, at work, and in other important areas of daily living. For example, someone with body dysmorphia may think that he or she has an unusually large nose (when it is really average size or only slightly large), and therefore avoids or reduces time spent at social occasions or work.

If you meet the criteria for any of these psychological conditions, then you shouldn't seek the solution to your problems through cosmetic surgery. Instead, consider seeking counseling to treat the disorder—they are all treatable, and you will feel so much better about yourself, without cosmetic surgery, once you get help.

When Cosmetic Surgery Is Right for You

OK, so you've ruled out any and all possibilities that your problem is psychological, and you have determined that you are right for cosmetic surgery. Now it's time to decide if cosmetic surgery is right for you! Let's take a closer look at your physical health, your lifestyle, and your schedule. If all three are conducive to surgery, then you're ready to go!

Are You Healthy?

What's your health status like? Are you in reasonably good health? Make an appointment with your physician to get a checkup if you haven't had one recently.

Do you have any kind of chronic illnesses that might complicate your surgery or any kind of physical ailment that might be made worse by going ahead with your cosmetic operation? If you do suffer from chronic illness or any kind of physical ailment, talk with your medical doctor before seeing a cosmetic surgeon, and get his or her opinion about whether or not cosmetic surgery is right for you. If you suffer from untreated lung or heart disease, untreated diabetes, or uncontrolled high blood pressure, cosmetic surgery may not be an appropriate option for you.

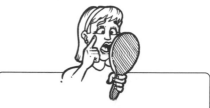

Wrinkle Ahead!

Discuss your health status and your desire for plastic surgery with your physician before seeking a consultation with a cosmetic surgeon.

Does Cosmetic Surgery Make Sense with Your Lifestyle?

Once you've had a checkup and received approval from your physician to seek consultation for cosmetic surgery, it's time to take a close look at your lifestyle. Some activities that could complicate your surgery or have a less-than-desirable effect on its final results include:

➤ smoking.

➤ frequent consumption of alcohol.

➤ recreational drug use.

➤ spending a lot of time outside without sunscreen.

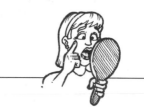

Wrinkle Ahead!

Don't cheat when it comes to smoking and surgery. If your doctor tells you to quit smoking before having a procedure, then do it! The nicotine in your system can greatly increase the risk of several side effects, including poor circulation and skin death. It's not worth it!

Engaging in any of these activities can complicate your surgery and produce unfavorable effects on your appearance. Be prepared to stop practicing these activities before, during, and after your surgery in order to ensure that your surgery will have the desired effects.

Do You Have the Time for a Cosmetic Procedure?

As you know by now, there is a wide variety of cosmetic procedures that you can choose from to help you improve your appearance. While some of these involve very little or no recovery time, others involve weeks or even months of recovery and follow-up treatment. Even if you have a clean bill of health and live the right kind of lifestyle, you may find that you're not in a position to take the time off of work or away from your family that the surgery you desire requires.

In the following chapters we provide an estimate of how much recovery time each cosmetic procedure involves. It's important to be aware of these requirements and to make the time in your schedule for the surgery. Is it feasible for you to take time off work or away from your other daily responsibilities to undergo a procedure?

If you elect a procedure that requires surgery, you will need to take a minimum of two weeks vacation in order to ensure a complete and safe recovery. Don't forget that you will need someone to care for you after your operation, as you should not be left unattended. Also, under no circumstances should you drive or operate any kind of machinery (like exercise equipment) during your recovery period. You'll be reminded of these facts throughout this book, and more details about these two subjects will be discussed in Chapter 28, "Taking Care of Yourself."

Do you think you're ready for cosmetic surgery? Take this quiz to find out for sure.

The Cosmetic Surgery Readiness Quiz

1. Do you think that cosmetic surgery will solve your life's difficulties or improve the quality of your life?
   Yes____   No____

2. Do you think that you will like yourself better after surgery?
   Yes____   No____

3. Do you see your body the way that other people do?
   Yes____   No____

4. Do you think you might have a distorted body image?
   Yes____   No____

5. Do you usually feel unhappy or depressed?
   Yes____   No____

---

6. Do you usually experience feelings of emptiness or irritability?
   Yes____   No____

7. Have you recently lost interest in pleasurable activities like hobbies or sex?
   Yes____   No____

8. Have you recently lost or gained more than 10 pounds?
   Yes____   No____

9. Have you recently begun sleeping more or less?
   Yes____   No____

10. Do you frequently tend to feel guilty?
    Yes____   No____

11. Do you feel hopeless or worthless?
    Yes____   No____

12. Do you have a tendency to binge or overeat?
    Yes____   No____

13. Do you ever engage in purging behaviors like skipping meals, excessive exercise, misuse of diuretics or laxatives, or self-induced vomiting?
    Yes____   No____

14. Are you unusually overweight?
    Yes____   No____

15. Do you smoke?
    Yes____   No____

16. Do you drink alcohol?
    Yes____   No____

17. Do you use drugs recreationally?
    Yes____   No____

18. Do you spend a lot of time in the sun?
    Yes____   No____

19. Do you suffer from heart or lung disease or diabetes?
    Yes____   No____

20. Do you suffer from any other chronic ailments?
    Yes____   No____

If you answered yes to any of these questions, a trip to your psychologist's or medical doctor's office may be in order before you pursue any avenue of cosmetic surgery. Be sure to rule out any psychological problems or medical problems before scheduling any kind of elective surgery. You'll end up being much happier with your results, if you do indeed decide to have surgery.

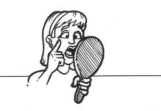

Wrinkle Ahead!

No cheating! An honest evaluation means taking a realistic view of what your face (without makeup) and body (without clothes and without sucking in your stomach) look like in natural light. Assessing your appearance with full makeup in a half-lit room with soft lighting from two feet away from the mirror will not allow you to form a realistic opinion of what needs improvement.

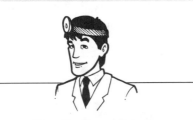

The Doctors Are In

Focus on one body part to improve at a time unless your doctor considers them to be minor procedures or major surgeries that are safe to have performed together. Having more than one major operation performed at the same time requires lengthy anesthesia, and that can increase the chances of complications or discomfort after surgery.

Defining the Problem

After you have unequivocally decided that you are right for cosmetic surgery and that cosmetic surgery is right for you, you'll need to determine what aspects of your appearance you wish to improve the most. In order to do that, you must evaluate your body with utter honesty. This means taking a good long look in the mirror—up close and from many different angles—to determine what body parts you want to improve and how you want to improve them. You can do this by undressing and looking at yourself in a full-length mirror, or by holding a handheld mirror up to your face or other areas of your body that you are considering having surgically enhanced. Be sure to practice this self-evaluation exercise with the lights on or during daylight hours.

As you look in the mirror, choose one body part that bothers you the most. Just choose one, the one that you always seem to complain about to yourself when you look in the mirror to get ready for work, or the one you feel the most self-conscious about when you meet someone new. Then look at this body part up close in the mirror. Look at it from the front view, the side views, the top view, and the bottom view. Ask yourself what bothers you the most about this body part. Is it the shape? Is it the size? Is it too small or too big? Is it the texture? Is it too loose or too wrinkled? Is the skin discolored or of an uneven complexion?

Notice what it is exactly about this body part that you want to improve. Be specific! Repeat your self-evaluation a few days later. If you identify the same body part as the one most in need of improvement, then make enhancing this part of your body your cosmetic surgery goal.

It's important to keep in mind that your goal should be to improve your appearance, not completely change your looks. Your doctor can make you look better, but he can't make you 23, slim, and gorgeous if you're 50, overweight, and weren't even gorgeous at 23! Be realistic in your expectations.

After you have had at least six months to recover from your last procedure, you can try this exercise again to come up with a new goal if you feel it is necessary.

Knowing When to Say When

Knowing when to say when is essential when planning cosmetic surgery. Where do you draw the line between being an advocate of cosmetic surgery and becoming a cosmetic surgery addict? How much surgery is too much surgery? There are no easy answers, but there are a few general rules to keep in mind when determining where to draw the line and when to say when. Here are the Top Ten Rules for Saying "When" to Cosmetic Surgery …

1. When it endangers your physical health or safety.

2. When a number of doctors you have consulted do not recommend the procedure. Remember, no look is "to die for."

3. When you cannot afford to have the initial surgery done.

4. When you will be unable to pay for maintenance.

5. During any times of crisis (divorce, death of a loved one).

6. When you feel depressed or are suffering from a psychological condition.

7. When you begin to base your self-worth on your appearance.

8. When cosmetic surgery becomes an obsession or the most important thing in your life. For example, if you seem to spend most of your time and money on planning your next operation, it's time to say "when."

9. If your physical imperfections are "perfect imperfections" and do not bother you. Perfect imperfections are uncommon physical features that you like and make you unique, like Cindy Crawford's mole or the gap between David Letterman's teeth.

Write these rules down, and when you go to the cosmetic surgeon's office, don't leave home without them!

The Next Step

As you continue to determine if you are right for cosmetic surgery, a good rule of thumb is to remember that cosmetic surgery is for people who are in good mental, emotional, and physical health. After you have decided that you are right for cosmetic surgery and have sought proper consultation or have received adequate information, keep in mind that you are making this decision for yourself and not anybody else. You don't have to explain or justify your decisions to family members or friends if you don't want to.

The Least You Need to Know

➤ You're not ready for cosmetic surgery if you suffer from untreated emotional or psychological problems.

➤ Cosmetic surgery is right for you if you are in good health and have sufficient amounts of time and money.

➤ Be realistic about what cosmetic surgery can do for you.

➤ Make sure you know the signs of a cosmetic surgery addict and know how to avoid becoming one.

Chapter 3

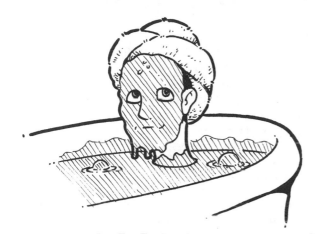

Nonsurgical Options

In This Chapter

➤ Finding the motivation to improve your beautiful self

➤ Nonsurgical options related to diet, exercise, and healthy lifestyle

➤ How smoking and other harmful practices affect how you look

➤ How to defy your aging process

If achieving the results of a cosmetic surgery appeal to you much more than actually having a cosmetic surgery performed, then you will be glad to learn that there are some cosmetic improvements that can be made without surgery. When electing to have any kind of cosmetic improvement made, it is important to know that there are two people who are responsible for creating any nonsurgical or surgical improvement to your appearance: your surgeon and you! Your surgeon is responsible for treating you, and you are responsible for protecting and maintaining the results of the treatment during your recovery period (if there is one) and beyond.

Once you are willing to take on the responsibility of maintaining your results, you are ready to learn about the three categories of nonsurgical options: diet and exercise, nonsurgical treatments and procedures, and medications and beauty supplements. These all can help you to achieve your cosmetic goals and look your absolute best.

Improving Beautiful Features Begins with Motivating Factors

Before you discover how to improve your beautiful features through the use of non-surgical techniques, it is important to develop an awareness of why you want to cosmetically improve your appearance. Whether you intend to use nonsurgical or surgical techniques in order to achieve your cosmetic goals, becoming aware of your motivating factors and being mindful of them before, during, and after your procedures will help you to accomplish your cosmetic goals and help you to be satisfied with your results. Most of all, an awareness of what motivated you to undergo a change will help you to stay committed to your decision to cosmetically improve your appearance at times when you are tempted to give up.

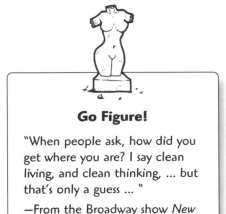

Go Figure!

"When people ask, how did you get where you are? I say clean living, and clean thinking, ... but that's only a guess ... "

—From the Broadway show *New Faces of 1956*

It is easy to abandon any new goal when you do not know or forget why you wanted to achieve it in the first place. Any achievement begins with at least one motivating factor. Without a consistent awareness of your own motivations, it is common for most people to let a busy schedule, a lack of energy, or any other surmountable obstacle prevent them from moving forward. They ultimately lose their ambition and fall short of accomplishing their goals. In these cases, excuses for failure quickly replace reasons for change.

In order to make you more likely to succeed in your goals, we would like to share with you some of the most common reasons why other people, many just like you, decide to cosmetically improve their appearance. See if the motivating factors below are some of the same reasons why you would like to cosmetically improve your appearance through nonsurgical techniques.

To Look the Same, Only Better

When some people decide to improve their appearance, they choose to look only slightly different after their procedure of choice is performed; they choose to look the same as they did before, only better. They already like the way that they look, they just want to have a subtle improvement made that will have a natural appearance and be undetectable to others once they have recovered from their procedure. For instance, some people might like the complexion and contour of their skin, but they may not like its texture. In this case, they would not choose to have a major surgery performed (such as a face-lift). Instead, they would elect to have a nonsurgical procedure performed in order to achieve their cosmetic goal of smoother and more radiant-looking skin. The result would be subtle and the procedure would be undetectable.

(See Chapter 25, "Get the Skin You Want Now! Soft-tissue Augmentation," for more details about nonsurgical options.)

To Delay the Appearance of Aging

Some men and women do not mind being of a certain age—they just do not want to look that age! For these men and women, any technique, especially a nonsurgical technique, that can improve their appearance is a very appealing option. Most nonsurgical alternatives can create a more youthful and vibrant appearance.

To Create a Feature Change

Some people have nonsurgical (and surgical) techniques performed to create a feature change. A feature change is an alteration of a major facial feature—such as an eye, a nose, or a lip—that completely changes the appearance of that feature. An example of a popular nonsurgical technique that can create a feature change is a collagen injection that can be made directly into a lip to improve shape and increase size. (See Chapter 25 for more details.)

To Create an Ethnic Change

An ethnic change is an alteration that is made to a feature of someone's appearance that is characteristic of a certain culture or ethnicity (like the larger-shaped noses that are characteristic of some Italian cultures or the wider-shaped noses of some African American cultures). This alteration is usually made surgically, but in some cases it can be created in a nonsurgical way. An example of a nonsurgical technique that can create an ethnic change is skin bleaching. Although we do not endorse this procedure (except to reduce the appearance of scars), many people of color do elect to have skin-bleaching treatments to lighten and brighten the color of their skin by a shade or two. In some cases, this can create the appearance of an ethnic change. Likewise, many people with naturally thin lips elect to have their lips enlarged through collagen injections or other procedures that alter the appearance of the lips that are naturally characteristic of their ethnicity. (Again, Chapter 25 offers more details about both of these procedures.)

To Feel Better

Some nonsurgical techniques that improve appearance are related to healthy eating and an active lifestyle. These kinds of diet- and exercise-related techniques (which will be described in greater detail in the next section of this chapter) can often prevent the physical signs of aging from appearing and can reduce feelings of sluggishness. Both are common reasons why people today are practicing nonsurgical techniques that are related to nutritious eating and a healthy and active lifestyle. After all, everyone wants to look and feel his or her best!

To Increase Energy

Some nonsurgical techniques that are related to diet and exercise can increase physical energy. They can have a weight-loss and electrolyte-balancing effect on the body that can produce greater amounts of physical energy. Just the endorphin rush that exercise creates can be a motivating factor for many people to practice some of the physical activities that fall under the category of nonsurgical techniques.

To Function More Effectively

It makes sense that when you experience an increase in physical energy, you can naturally function more effectively. Many people experience an increase in their ability to focus, can concentrate for longer periods of time, and can manage stress more easily when they have more energy. These are all benefits of increased physical energy, which is a result of healthy eating and exercise.

To Improve Productivity

Nonsurgical techniques that are related to diet, exercise, and supplements all tend to create more energy and empower people to function more effectively. As a further result, people also tend to improve their productivity levels when performing at work or performing daily activities at home. Is there any one of us who would not like to be more productive at work or at home?

To Prevent Disease

Nonsurgical alternatives that involve nutrition and an active lifestyle tend to be used not only as a method of preventing the appearance of aging, but also as a method of preventing disease. A healthy diet and exercise can reduce the risk of heart attack, stroke, and other medical problems from developing, or at least delay the onset of them for a significant period of time. Does this sound like a good motivating factor for you?

To Manage or Reduce Current Health Problems

Many of us tend to wait until the onset of physical symptoms of health problems to develop before we decide to change our unbalanced eating habits and sedentary lifestyle. If your doctor has warned you about any debilitating health problems that are related to diet or weight and you also would like to improve your appearance, a new regimen of balanced eating in addition to an active lifestyle may assist you in managing or reducing your current health problems. Talk to your doctor about whether or not he or she would recommend any of these changes in your daily living.

To Improve a Moderate Health Status

Some men and women who are interested in cosmetic surgery are not experiencing health problems and show no signs of any health risks. These are people in moderate health who just want to look and feel their absolute best. If this sounds like you, you might want to consider improving your condition from "moderate health" to an "excellent health" status.

To Live Longer

Many of us who have experienced a decline in our physical health, who are at risk for health problems, or who are over 50 years of age tend to be more aware of our health and mortality than those who have not had similar life experiences. If the familiar phrase "older and wiser" proves true, all of us will become more conscious of maintaining a moderate calorie intake and maintaining a healthy and active lifestyle as we grow older. These are two nonsurgical treatments that can help each of us to live as long as possible!

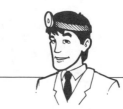

The Doctors Are In

Someone who is moderately healthy may have some health risk factors like being overweight but has not yet shown any acute symptoms like extremely high blood pressure or extremely high cholesterol levels (although they might have blood pressure levels and cholesterol levels that can be improved).

To Gain Attention

Another reason some of us seek out cosmetic improvements (both nonsurgical and surgical) is to gain attention from those around us. It is an unfair fact of life that most people are conditioned to notice and respond more favorably to an attractive-looking person. Our eyes naturally gravitate towards people who have an appearance that is aesthetically pleasing—they are like candy to the eyes.

Gaining the attention of others is a common motivating factor for some people to cosmetically improve their appearance. If this is one of your motivating factors, be sure you keep it in perspective and avoid letting it become your primary or sole reason for altering your appearance. If this is the case, you might need to see a psychologist instead of a surgeon. No one should feel the need to cosmetically alter his or her appearance at the whim of another person.

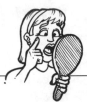

Wrinkle Ahead!

Those who have been conditioned to believe that attractive people usually receive more attention might turn to cosmetic surgery as a means to gain or keep the attention of those around them. Using cosmetic surgery of any kind for the sole purpose of gaining attention can be the first step down a very self-destructive path; their self-worth and the closeness of their relationships fluctuates with people's ever-changing definition of beauty and their own ever-changing appearance. Remember, as we age, our appearance is constantly evolving even if we don't alter it cosmetically. If the only reason you are choosing to alter your appearance is to get yourself noticed, know that there are less expensive and more effective types of attention-getting behavior that a skilled therapist could help you to discover and practice.

To Maintain Sexual Interest in a Relationship

There is no doubt that when cosmetic techniques are performed successfully, the results are attractive and can arouse sexual interest. Many women and men seek cosmetic procedures that will increase their sex appeal and keep sexual interest alive in their love relationships. As long as your love relationship and sex life are not primarily based on your appearance and/or whether or not you have a cosmetic technique performed, your relationship might benefit from a cosmetic procedure. Be certain that gaining or maintaining sexual interest is not the only reason for choosing a non-surgical technique. A psychologist or therapist can help you to keep this in healthy perspective.

To Receive Preferential Treatment

Everyone appreciates an attractive appearance. Most us have either witnessed or observed firsthand that if someone likes our appearance, we will most likely receive preferential treatment from that person. It is true that preferential treatment commonly comes with a preferred look. Attractive people are frequently favored over less attractive people for jobs, raises, and bonuses, and are given special allowances that are usually reserved for VIPs and the social elite.

To Avoid Having a Major Surgery Performed Later

It seems to be a medical fact that if you have minor cosmetic procedures performed along the way, there tends to be less of a need for major cosmetic surgeries to be performed later in life. One reason for this could be that when you have skin, fat, or tissue removed or revised when it initially becomes problematic, it does not have a chance to put pressure on surrounding areas of the body and cause them to sag downward along with it or to lose their natural shape. An ounce of prevention is often worth a pound of cure! Several minor nonsurgical procedures over time can often produce the same results as a major surgery.

To Save Money

Minor nonsurgical procedures tend to be less expensive than major cosmetic surgeries, depending on which procedure is performed. The large discrepancy in price is due to the requirement for general anesthesia. Unlike most major cosmetic surgeries, nonsurgical procedures do not require general anesthesia (only local anesthesia for some procedures). Many people would rather pay a smaller price for an occasional minor procedure to prevent signs of aging from developing instead of paying a larger price for a major cosmetic surgery to repair or conceal signs of aging that develop later in life.

Now that you've read this list of motivational factors, can you think of any other reasons that might motivate you to have a cosmetic procedure performed? Try to think of as many as you can. We recommend that you write them down on a piece of paper and keep the list in a place where you can easily read it before and after your cosmetic procedure. It will help you to remember what your motivations are for improving your appearance. Keep these factors in mind, especially when you feel like giving up on a procedure that will benefit you. Staying focused will help you to maintain your ambition and to achieve your cosmetic goals.

Quick Fixes vs. Long-Term Goals

Nonsurgical techniques are procedures that do not require surgery. In other words, they do not require incisions to be placed in the skin or for the skin to be broken in any way (except when needles are used for a technique that require an injection). Most nonsurgical techniques do not require a recovery period or any down time, and the results are immediate.

With most nonsurgical techniques, the effects are only permanent if you maintain them through proper care and/or repeated treatments. For this

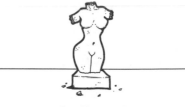

Go Figure!

Nonsurgical options work better as methods of preventing the signs of aging from developing rather than treatment for the signs that already exist. Many nonsurgical techniques can postpone a need for cosmetic surgery, while only few can replace it.

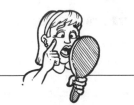

Wrinkle Ahead!

Although nonsurgical techniques are considered quick fixes, major cosmetic surgery can also be considered a quick fix for the signs of aging if you have smoked, drank alcohol, and spent much of your daily living outside in the sun, and continue to do so after your surgery. Remember, any cosmetic result can be lost almost as quickly as it has been achieved!

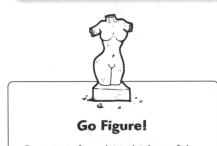

Go Figure!

Protein is found in chicken, fish, most white meats, and egg whites. Carbohydrates are found in breads, pastas, potatoes, rice, and grains. Dairy products consist of milk, cheese, and eggs. Fruits you can eat are bananas, apples, oranges, grapes, pears, melons, strawberries, and so on. Some vegetables you might want to include in your diet are green leafy vegetables like spinach and salad, carrots, peas, and squash.

reason, nonsurgical techniques are usually considered to be quick fixes, and major surgical techniques produce more permanent results. However, if you have any cosmetic procedure performed (surgical or nonsurgical), the results will last only for as long as you protect them with proper care.

The foundation for the success of any cosmetic procedure, including a nonsurgical technique, is your biological predisposition and the condition of your body at the time of your treatment. In other words, whatever body Mother Nature gave you at birth, how you have treated it over the years, and the condition that it is in when you have your cosmetic procedure performed will be what you and your surgeon will have to work with when you come in for treatment. For example, if you have a genetic predisposition toward being overweight or if you have gained excessive amounts of weight from overeating, a heavy body will be the foundation for your procedure. If you have maintained an average body weight and avoided the damaging rays of the sun, a lean structure with skin that is free from sun damage will be the basic structure for your treatment. It is what you and your doctor have to work with. The current condition of your body will be what your surgeon will be in charge of treating and what you will be in charge of healing.

Most nonsurgical techniques are alternatives that are best used to prevent the development of the signs of aging rather than treatment for the telltale signs of aging that have already appeared. Many of the nonsurgical options that produce cosmetic improvements pertain to diet and a healthy and active lifestyle.

Eat Well-Balanced Meals

Eat well-balanced meals that give you your USDA daily requirements of protein, carbohydrates, dairy, fruits, vegetables, and fats. A total daily caloric intake for the average person is about 2,000 calories. The intake can be less if the person is smaller (due to bone structure, not weight) than average, or more if the person is larger than average size.

Eat Regularly and Moderately

Eat regularly and moderately throughout the day. You can divide your daily calorie intake into three to five small meals, which will fuel your system and give you adequate calories for energy throughout the day. This also regulates your metabolism and keeps it burning calories on a regular basis. When your metabolism is regulated, it burns calories more easily. Keep that in mind and avoid starving yourself to lose or maintain weight. You will get better results if you feed your system the food that it needs regularly and moderately.

Take Vitamins and Minerals

When your nutritional needs are met, you will be less likely to want to overeat. Frequently it is a mineral deficiency, not a calorie deficiency, that propels many people to experience cravings and to overeat. Minerals are present in your multiple vitamins and some protein powders. Drop by your local drugstore, pharmacy, or health-food store and pick up a multi-vitamin of your choice. Also, know that B Complex with B12 and folic acid seems to have a protective element that can help to prevent vascular disease. Be sure to put these on your shopping list when you go to your local drugstore!

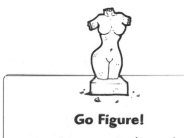

Go Figure!

Vitamins including A (retinol), B, C, and E can help to keep you looking young! Retinol, if applied to the skin, has a profoundly good effect on skin. A little C helps build collagen, but too much inhibits it.

Drink Plenty of Water

Your body is made up of more than 60 percent water. The majority of your entire physical being consists of and needs water in order to sustain itself in a healthy manner. Yet most of us do not drink our daily requirement of six to eight 8-ounce glasses of water each day. Consider this fact and be sure to drink your daily requirement.

Don't Smoke

Smoking can cause severe health problems such as emphysema and lung cancer. One of its less serious but equally damaging effects is prematurely wrinkled skin. Smoking constricts your blood vessels and causes the skin to wrinkle. If you want your skin to look its best for as long as it can, avoid or quit smoking!

Avoid Drinking Alcohol

There are many health risks that chronic consumption of alcohol poses. Other than the life-threatening liver conditions that it can cause, it can also cause you to gain unwanted weight. Remember, excess weight can pull your skin and surrounding tissue downward, causing needless sagging and drooping to occur. In addition, chronic alcohol consumption robs your skin's system of the necessary elements to keep itself looking young and fresh. For the sake of your health and appearance, we recommend that you avoid or quit drinking alcohol.

Avoid Recreational Drug Use

Aside from the obvious fact that use of recreational drugs (including marijuana without a prescription) is illegal and punishable by law, it also poses many serious health risks. It robs your body of its natural elements and impairs normal functioning that can easily lend itself to needless accidents and disaster. (In males, it decreases testosterone levels and amphetamine-like drugs constrict blood vessels.) It can also create a host of internal and external damages over a long period of time, and an overdose of any recreational drug can result in almost immediate death or permanent disability.

The least of its effects is a poor quality of color, complexion, contour, and elasticity of your skin. It also does not mix well with medications (including anesthesia) that you will be given during and after your surgery. Strangely, this last result is often the only motivating factor that some people choose to avoid recreational drug use. Your reason for avoiding recreational drugs really doesn't matter, but we do encourage you to choose one, even if it is the preservation of your beautiful appearance.

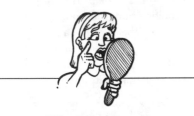

Wrinkle Ahead!

You really can delay or prevent the need for cosmetic surgery. A lot of what causes aging is related to behavior that produces wear and tear on the body. There are those who are genetically protected, but this protection is not indefinite. The wear and tear is related to the oxidation from a number of popular vices or activities such as eating, sunning, drinking alcohol, and being exposed to irritants such as cigarette smoke and atmospheric oxidants.

Avoid Damaging Rays of the Sun

By avoiding sun exposure, you will protect your skin from sun damage. Sun damage is characterized by skin that appears to have aged prematurely due to chronic sun exposure. The signs of premature aging that results from chronic sun exposure are an uneven, blotchy, or spotted complexion, loss of elasticity, thickening of the skin, and sagging or drooping of the skin. Do any of these effects sound like a good price to pay for a year-round tan to you?

Exercise Regularly

Weight maintenance through cardiovascular exercise (walking, jogging, biking, swimming) can improve the function of your cardiovascular system, which is partially responsible for the transportation of oxygen through your blood stream and for the flow of blood throughout your entire body. Improving your cardiovascular functioning can prevent the development of health problems like heart attack and stroke, and improve your overall health.

Maintain a Healthy and Stable Weight

If you lose excess weight or maintain a healthy weight, you can put less pressure on your body and can spare your organs and joints from the unnecessary demands of excess weight. There will be less weight for your body to carry, so it will suffer less wear. Also, keep in mind that only about 10 percent of your weight is blood. So, if you weigh less, your blood can travel through your body much easier and cardiovascular functioning can be improved!

Get Plenty of Rest

When your body is it at rest, it begins to heal itself and to recover from the wear and tear of the day. Without sufficient rest, your body does not have the opportunity to perform its necessary repairs. Its natural healing process is interrupted and delayed. If you want to look your absolute best without surgery, be sure to get six to eight hours of sleep each night. This will help your body to recover from the day, make any necessary repairs, and help you to feel refreshed and look vibrant the next day.

Also, if you don't already have a regular bedtime, start one now! Irregular and minimal sleep patterns can place extra stress on your body and can prevent you from looking your best. They call it "beauty rest" for a very good reason!

Review these nonsurgical tips to improve your general health and outward appearance. Consistent use of these techniques will help to keep you feeling good and looking great! We will also remind you of these nonsurgical techniques anytime they apply to different surgeries described throughout the chapters in this book.

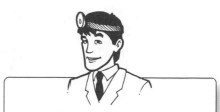

The Doctors Are In

Use it or lose it! The exercised body stimulates hormones that maintain the body's vitality. The larger muscles that are activated during consistent exercise speed up the resting metabolism and help you to maintain a healthy weight. Take care of your body and your body will take care of you!

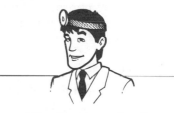

The Doctors Are In

When you are tempted to overeat or make a meal out of unhealthy snack foods, visualize where on your body you would place the fat from the food you are eating. This may help motivate you to eat more nutritious foods and to eat more moderately.

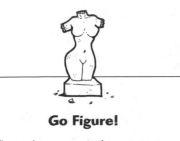

Mother's Little Helpers

Some of us who seek out cosmetic improvements, whether surgical or nonsurgical, have already treated our bodies with proper nutrition and exercise. We have avoided smoking, drinking, and recreational drug use, and have even maintained active lifestyles that include a healthy amount of exercise. However, the bodies that Mother Nature gave us haven't responded as favorably as we would have liked to these techniques and seem to need just a little bit more help. We have already determined that cosmetic improvements need to be made but we do not want to endure the pain and other costs of surgical treatment. For those of us in this condition, there are other noninvasive procedures that are considered to be nonsurgical treatments.

The most popular and effective nonsurgical treatments available for facial improvements are listed below. Remember that nutritional eating and maintaining an active and healthy lifestyle are the only nonsurgical treatments that can improve the shape of your body. All other cosmetic improvements require surgery.

Facials

Facials are nonsurgical treatments that cleanse, tone, and moisturize the face. The products used during this procedure are as varied as the practitioners who perform them. Facials can reduce the appearance of fine lines and wrinkles by temporarily tightening and toning your skin. They can be performed in a dermatologist's office, spa, or beauty salon.

There are also over-the-counter products that you can buy to perform your facial treatment in the comfort of your own home. The results are temporary and last only if they are maintained through repeated monthly treatments.

Salon facials vary in strength and are priced accordingly. Most salon facials start at anywhere between $50 and $100 and go up from there.

Galvanic Current

Galvanic current began in the 1920s and was used to treat and reduce the appearance of preexisting wrinkles. An electric current was applied directly to fine lines and wrinkles through an instrument that would eventually evolve into an applicator of many different shapes and sizes that practitioners use today. The application of this current to the skin resulted in temporary swelling that would reduce the appearance of fine lines and wrinkles. It remains a short-term treatment that carries with it the possibility of long-term scars if it is misused. Although it is not the treatment of choice for the smart man or woman today and it is not a treatment that we highly recommend, it is a nonsurgical option that is still available today for the average price of $100 or more per session.

Check out the soft-tissue augmentation chapter in this book (Chapter 25) for many, many more nonsurgical options! And, as we say in the beauty business, "No list is ever complete!" Continue to watch for new and exciting cosmetic advancements in the field of medicine such as medications, nonsurgical treatments and therapies, and appearance-altering operations. New ones are being developed all the time.

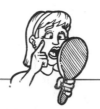

Wrinkle Ahead!

Facial exercises are a popular but counter-productive technique for preventing or reducing the appearance of wrinkles. Performing facial exercises over an extended period of time will actually contribute to the development of facial lines. If you think about it for a moment, when you exercise your abdomen, you develop horizontal lines that cross the natural vertical lines of your abdomen and create a "six-pack" appearance. If you exercise your neck muscles, forehead muscles, or smile lines, the muscular enlargement will cause facial lines to develop and call attention to any facial lines that already exist. Facial lines from exercises can develop perpendicular to wrinkle lines!

Defying Your Aging Process

Even if you practice the nonsurgical techniques related to diet, exercise, and healthy living, and you take care of your skin with facial treatments, your body still might not respond as well as you would like. If your body does not respond as favorably to these nonsurgical techniques, you may be experiencing *hormonal failure*. This condition affects all areas of the body and can only be treated medically. The other nonsurgical treatments that we have already mentioned can assist in your treatment of hormonal failure, but they cannot adequately remedy the problem by themselves.

When hormonal failure occurs, most people experience these common symptoms:

➤ Slower metabolism

➤ Weight gain

➤ Loss of skin elasticity (results in drooping, sagging, and wrinkling of the skin)

➤ Lack of physical energy

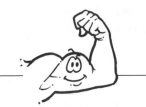

➤ Hair loss

➤ A less vibrant complexion

These are the most common symptoms that are problematic for people who look to cosmetic surgery as a remedy for the physical results of hormonal failure. Surgery can clean up some of the physical results of hormonal failure, but it cannot adequately delay the actual aging process.

Better Definition

Hormonal failure is mainly characterized by a reduction in available testosterone levels in men and a decrease in the estrogen levels in women. Hormonal failure is a natural development that occurs as we age, and some people experience hormonal failure earlier and at a more rapid pace than others.

Hormone-replacement therapy is the only nonsurgical treatment that can actually delay a part of the aging process and its appearance. Hormone-replacement therapy is a relatively new idea that replaces the main hormones that your body has lost as it has aged. This therapy restores hormone levels to that of a younger person. This can help some major symptoms of hormonal failure by either enhancing your current physical state or by delaying the outward appearances of the aging process.

The most popular substances used to treat the effects of hormonal failure are estrogen, testosterone, and HGH. All of these are commonly used to treat the results of aging, but not all of these substances would necessarily be considered a hormone-replacement therapy by all physicians' standards. However, they are the most important nonsurgical treatments that many people ask their doctor for when making cosmetic improvements to counter the effects of hormonal failure.

Estrogen

Estrogen and its analogues come typically as a topical estrogen cream, and ingestible pills. Other medications and creams may also contain derivatives of estrogen. Women can usually benefit from one or all of these treatments. A topical estrogen cream can also moisturize and smooth out the top layer of the skin in both men and women.

Ingestible or injectable estrogen will hormonally balance a woman's body if she is experiencing any symptoms of hormonal failure. It can also help to reduce or eliminate the mood swings and hot flashes that often accompany menopause. Early treatments of estrogen can delay the onset of menopause. In many cases, estrogen is needed on an ongoing basis in order to counterbalance the ongoing effects of hormonal failure.

Talk with your doctor to see if you could benefit from a few regular doses of hormonal replacement therapy. It can improve your body from the inside out and is available only by prescription. Prices vary depending on the form and dose of estrogen that is needed.

Testosterone

Testosterone is most safely used as a typical cream form as a hormone-replacement therapy for men. There are also other analogues of testosterone, including patches, ointments, and lozenges. New analogues are developing and will be released soon. Most men report a noticeable increase in physical strength and energy from testosterone injections. In some cases, men can experience a mild depression that can mimick the emotional ups and downs of PMS if the correct dosage has not been determined. It is common for a doctor to experiment with different dosages until the patient responds favorably. Women who have unusually low doses of estrogen can also benefit from this type of hormone-replacement therapy.

HGH or Somatotropin

HGH is an injectable hormone-replacement therapy that has been available for the last 10 years but has only recently received much attention as an anti-aging technique. HGH (human growth hormone) or somatotropin is the rebuilding hormone that can cause redistribution of fat in a more favorable way. It can cause leaner muscle mass and decreases fat. It increases bone density and may increase immunity.

Somatotropin can also have adverse side effects that may be permanent. Overly large doses that are misused over a long period of time could result in the development of a protruding forehead, enlarged jaw, enlarged hands or wrists, enlarged fingers, increased blood sugar, increased blood pressure, and headaches. If there is a risk of cancer it is not known at this time. It is a very controversial anti-aging strategy because long-term effects of its use are still undetermined. It usually takes about 20 years for medical experts to determine a treatment's effectiveness and its safety.

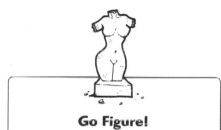

Go Figure!

The first classic sign of hormonal failure is the development of fat above the belly button in the male and below the belly button in the female. Females also develop fatty arms and thighs. The midsection and the texture of the skin also frequently become softer and flabby. Hormone-replacement therapy is the answer to this dilemma—not liposuction. Even if you have liposuction performed, you must still have hormonal replacement therapy if you have hormonal failure.

Finistride

Finistride (also known as Propecia or Proscar) is used widely to treat male-pattern baldness in men. Testosterone breaks down into DHT (DHT, or di-hydroxy-testosterone) and DHT causes hair loss and an increase in fat in the abdomen. Finistride blocks the delivery of DHT to the scalp, where it would normally cause hair loss if its travel plans were not interrupted. The intervention of finistride helps to prevent the loss of hair, and in many cases can even stimulate hair regrowth in the crown area of the head.

We recommend that you carefully consider these nonsurgical techniques. Currently, they have all proven themselves to be effective in either slowing down the aging process and/or improving your appearance to a very satisfactory degree. They are all effective strategies for looking your best, and none of them require surgery.

Beauty Supplements

Many over-the-counter beauty products contain active ingredients that will enhance the results of the other nonsurgical techniques discussed above. They are all rejuvenating elements that your skin naturally contains. The following active ingredients found in some beauty supplements can coax your skin into smoothing out and contracting into a more youthful position:

➤ **Hyaluronic acid:** Hydronic acid is present in the skin and helps to keep moisture in the skin. You are born with large amounts of this in your skin and it diminishes as you age. It can be passively absorbed if it is applied to the skin by applying a cream or moisturizer that contains this ingredient.

➤ **Mucopolysaccharides:** Mucopolysaccharides are also a natural component of the skin. They can be passively absorbed through creams and moisturizers as well. They are a natural part of your body's normal moisturizing system and have some antibacterial effects.

➤ **NaPCA:** NaPCA is a natural moisturizer of the skin. It comes in a liquid form over the counter and can be sprayed on your face. It is easily absorbed and might aid in keeping your face smooth and supple.

➤ **Zinc:** Zinc can promote collagen reproduction. Collagen is a natural ingredient in the skin that is partially responsible for skin elasticity. Zinc also is an antibacterial/antifungal agent that helps to keep your skin looking clean and fresh.

➤ **Cell stimulators:** Cell stimulators come in many forms. They can be enzymes or stimulating proteins that act as keys in a lock, turning on certain cell functions that normally would not be turned on by the body anymore. This can stimulate collagen to grow, which in turn promotes skin elasticity and reduces the skin's tendency to scar; it can even improve the appearance of preexisting scars. Cell stimulators are found in one over-the-counter product today called Return.

Using a variety of the techniques discussed in this chapter in conjunction with each other can keep you in great shape for a longer period of time and might delay the need for any cosmetic surgery. If cosmetic surgery is needed, your surgery will certainly be easier to perform and your recovery period will go more smoothly because your body will be in prime condition for surgery.

The Least You Need to Know

➤ A healthy diet, exercise, and the avoidance of smoking, recreational drug use (including marijuana), alcohol use, and chronic sun exposure are all nonsurgical techniques that can improve your appearance.

➤ Facials are the No. 1 treatment of choice for smart men and women who want to nonsurgically improve their appearance by having an actual procedure performed.

➤ Hormone-replacement therapy is a very popular nonsurgical treatment.

➤ Many over-the-counter beauty supplements contain active ingredients that can nonsurgically improve your appearance!

Chapter 4

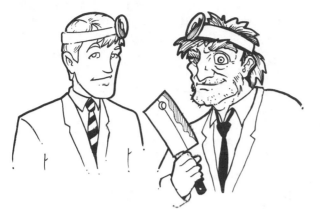

Choosing a Doctor Who's Right for You

In This Chapter

➤ What everyone should know about his or her doctor

➤ How to take charge of your surgery

➤ Idiot-proof tips for selecting the right doctor

➤ How to prepare for your consult

If you're daunted by the task of choosing the right doctor for your cosmetic procedure, you're not alone! Thousands of people seek cosmetic surgery every year in the United States and Canada, and a vast majority of them are apprehensive and confused by the process of selecting an appropriate physician.

Finding a cosmetic surgeon who has perfected his or her surgical skills and who is affordable is just as important as finding someone you can trust to give you the quality of care that you deserve. The information in this chapter will help you to decipher between the doctors who are right for someone else and the doctor who is right for you!

What You Should Know About Your Doctor

Before you entrust a doctor with your appearance, you should make sure he or she is qualified and experienced. In this section, we'll review the most basic criteria any doctor should meet before you agree to have him or her perform a procedure.

Board Certification

Medical licenses allow doctors to practice a wide range of surgery, including cosmetic surgery, even if they have not had extensive training in this area. For example, it is legally possible for any M.D. to take a weekend class on cosmetic surgery, advertise himself or herself as a cosmetic surgeon, and then perform a cosmetic procedure of your choice on you!

The only way you can be absolutely certain that a doctor has had extensive training in cosmetic surgery is if he or she is certified by the American Board of Plastic Surgery (ABPS) or is a member of the American Society of Plastic and Reconstructive Surgeons (ASPRS). Doctors must meet extensive requirements in order to be certified by the ABPS or to become members of ASPRS.

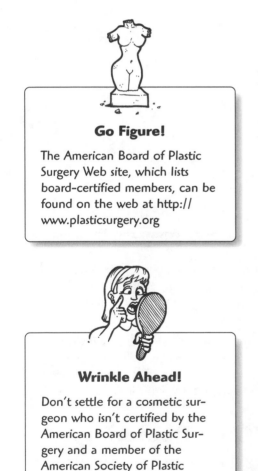

Go Figure!

The American Board of Plastic Surgery Web site, which lists board-certified members, can be found on the web at http://www.plasticsurgery.org

Wrinkle Ahead!

Don't settle for a cosmetic surgeon who isn't certified by the American Board of Plastic Surgery and a member of the American Society of Plastic Surgeons.

Track Record

Once you have ascertained that a doctor is certified by the ABPS, it's time to check his or her track record. You can do this by asking the medical board of the state that the doctor is operating in the following questions:

➤ Is the doctor licensed to operate in that state?

➤ Have there been any malpractice suits filed against him or her?

➤ Has any disciplinary action ever been taken against the physician?

➤ Is he or she on probation, or has he or she ever been on probation?

You have a right to know all of these things about each doctor you meet before you determine which one is right for you.

Don't Become a Guinea Pig!

After you've screened for credentials and a good track record, you can move on to the physician's surgical skills. Ask your doctor if he or she specializes in the procedure you want to have performed, whether it be a breast enlargement or a tummy tuck. Find out how many of these procedures he or she has performed.

Make sure that the doctor is experienced in the procedure you are seeking. The last thing you want is a doctor who has just finished a weekend class on the subject and is looking forward to having you as his or her first patient. You don't want to be anyone's guinea pig!

It may feel uncomfortable for you to ask these questions, but do it anyway. Remember, your appearance and your life depend on the questions you ask—as well as the questions you don't ask.

Taking Charge of Your Surgery

You must thoroughly interview each doctor you're considering having perform your surgery. This might involve meetings with several different doctors, and you'll need to know the right questions to ask during your consultation. This can be a real challenge if you've never had a cosmetic procedure performed or feel intimidated by doctors. We recognize this challenge, and have written the next segment in order to help you take charge of your surgery, feel more relaxed, and gather all the information you'll need from each board-certified surgeon that you consider selecting.

Idiot-Proof Tips for Selecting the Right Doctor

> ➤ State what physical feature you would like cosmetically improved and why. Suggest a procedure and ask for your doctor's recommendation. For instance, you might say, "I don't like these wrinkles around my eyes because they make me look older than I am. I'd like to have surgery on my upper lids." He or she might agree with diminishing the appearance of the wrinkles but may suggest another alternative that might be more effective, like collagen injections.

> ➤ Ask your doctor what can go *wrong* instead of *right* with the recommended surgery. Learn the common and uncommon risks of the surgery. Don't be swayed by the hype of a new procedure or the enthusiasm of your doctor. Find out the facts and consider the risks. You have a right to make a fully informed decision.

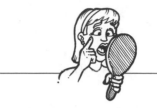

Wrinkle Ahead!

Watch out for advertisements that indicate a cosmetic surgeon is "board certified" but which don't specify what kind of board it is—there are lots of boards out there offering certification, but only the American Board of Plastic Surgery is recognized by the American Board of Medical Specialties.

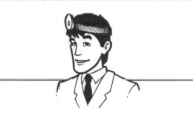

The Doctors Are In

Make sure you feel comfortable with the physician and that you feel you can trust him or her. Even if a doctor is completely qualified to perform a procedure, if you don't feel comfortable with him or her, there is a greater chance that you'll be dissatisfied with the final outcome of your procedure.

➤ Ask your doctor about alternative surgeries or nonsurgical solutions to remedy the physical feature you would like to have improved.

➤ Ask your doctor for information about the recommended procedure and study it carefully at home. What is a typical result from such a procedure? Is maintenance surgery going to be required later on? If so, how much later?

➤ Ask if any of the staff has had surgery and find out how their procedure was.

➤ Find out who the best candidates are for this procedure. People of different colors, ages, and ethnicities can heal differently or may be at greater risk for certain complications. Make sure you would be a good candidate for the procedure.

➤ Find out exactly how the surgery is performed. Ask your doctor to explain it to you step-by-step so you know what to expect. You don't want to wake up to any surprises after your surgery; you should know ahead of time what you will look and feel like after your operation. Address with your doctor how the incisions will be closed (with stitches or sutures) and the pros and cons of each alternative.

➤ Make sure you know where the surgery will take place. Some doctors have in-office operating rooms, while others utilize space at other doctor's offices or hospitals. Ask to see the operating room. Inspect it for cleanliness and ask your doctor if it is fully equipped with proper instruments in case of a life-threatening emergency or any other crisis. Not all operating rooms come fully equipped to handle some accidents. Most hospital operating rooms are fully equipped for such emergencies. Be sure that your surgeons operating room is fully-equipped and certified by a reputable agency like AAAAP or JACH.

➤ Ask who will be performing the entire surgery. Sometimes doctors have their assistants take over the operation after a surgery has begun. Be sure that your doctor will either perform the entire surgery or be present during the entire operation.

Bonus tip:

➤ Last, but not least, document everything! Take a journal with you and write down all of your questions and the answers of each doctor that you interviewed. Otherwise, all of your valuable information, if left up to memory, could be lost. Also, you'll want to have a written record noting the date of the interview and what responses each doctor gave to your questions. This will give you peace of mind and prevent any future confusion about what was actually said if there is a problem later on with your surgery. If you didn't write down the details of your interview with the doctor, it will be difficult to remember what was said and how the doctors opinions differ.

There you have it! These are the most important questions to consider when selecting a doctor that's right for you. But wait! There are a few other things you'll want to take into consideration before making your final decision.

Things to Bring Up During Your Consult

You can never be too thorough when it comes to considering all of the factors involved in cosmetic surgery. They are as numerous as they are important, and each one requires exquisite care. Take your time when selecting a surgeon and consider everything that the surgery will require of you before, during, and after your operation.

Here are a few more things to consider before placing your trust and your ultimate appearance in a physician's hands:

When can you return to your normal, everyday routine?

Different surgeries require different lengths of recovery time. Your recovery time will depend on how minor or major of a surgery was performed, what muscles or tissues were cut during your operation, how your body responds to surgery as well as how it heals, and if there were any complications involved during or after your operation.

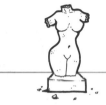

Go Figure!

An initial consult with a cosmetic surgeon might be free or it might cost as much as $175—the fee varies from area to area and cosmetic surgeon to cosmetic surgeon.

For surgeries that don't seem too complex like scar reduction or liposuction, you can return to work in just a few days. Major surgeries like face-lifts or calf implants can take weeks, possibly even months, to completely heal, especially if there are complications (like an infection) involved. Ask your doctor how long it will be before you can return to your normal, everyday routine (work, gym, sexual activity, and so on).

When will you see your final results?

It will take awhile before you can see the final results of your surgery. Different surgeries have different recovery times, so the point at which you can see your final results will vary. For instance, if you have a face-lift or your eyes done, the contour of your face and eyes will change over a period of one to three months, although most of the bruising and swelling will be gone in a matter of weeks. If your surgery is more minor, like liposuction, final results can be seen in just a few weeks.

Ask your doctor when you can expect to see the final results of your surgery … and be patient! Sometimes people insist that their surgery did not give them the results that they wanted when they really haven't given themselves time enough to heal or effectively talked about post-operative healing with the doctor.

53

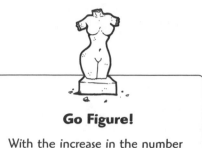

How can you camouflage the fact that you've had surgery?

For some people, this is a very important question because, while they want to improve their appearance, they want the results to look natural without revealing to the whole world that they have indeed had surgical assistance. To others, this is less important. It is easier for women to disguise their surgery with makeup, hats, scarves, large sunglasses, and other accessories.

It is more difficult for men to camouflage their surgery unless a baseball hat, a high-collared shirt (like a turtleneck), or large ski glasses are in season and will adequately cover the surgical area. If they are not, these accessories may draw attention and solicit questions from people. If concealing the fact that you've had surgery is important to you, ask your doctor how you can best camouflage your incisions.

Go Figure!

With the increase in the number of people having cosmetic procedures, fewer people care whether others know they are having a cosmetic improvement made. It's a personal decision, though, and you should only tell people about it if you feel comfortable with others knowing.

What happens if a revision is needed?

A revision is a touch-up surgery that doctors perform at their patient's request and cost, if the final results do not look aesthetically pleasing. Whether or not the results are "aesthetically pleasing" is a matter of opinion—your opinion!

It is uncommon for doctors and their patients to disagree over whether or not they received an acceptable result from their operation. Keeping this in mind, different doctors have different policies about revision and follow-up surgeries. Most if not all doctors usually require their patients to at least pay at a percentage of the costs of a revision surgery, or even to pay the entire amount.

Although revision surgeries are not frequently performed, they are usually considered to be a new and different surgery. Ask your doctor about his or her policy on revision surgeries and consider the possibility of these additional costs.

What will the total cost of your surgery be?

When you meet with your doctor, ask for an itemized list of the entire cost of your entire surgery from beginning to end. This would include preoperative visits, each surgery performed, anesthesia, all necessary and possible medications involved, and postoperative visits and care, as well as revision or follow-up surgeries.

You are entitled to know exactly how much your surgery is going to cost you. The last thing you'll want to worry about is money when you are recuperating. Your full-time job after your surgery will be just to get well and rest.

Will your doctor be available for aftercare?

Some doctors field aftercare responsibilities to other staff members, such as their assistants or nurses. This is a matter of concern for some patients because they feel like they are not being given the highest quality of care. They paid a high price for a service to be performed by their doctor, and they want their doctor to perform all duties of the operation from beginning to end, including aftercare.

Ask your doctor whether he or she will be available for aftercare and follow-up visits, or if you will be expected to see a nurse or another staff member. Consider whether or not you feel comfortable with your doctor's answer.

Refer to your journal and compare the answers of each surgeon to determine which doctor gave you answers that you liked the best. Take notice if their main concern was for your safety or if it was to have additional surgeries done that are really not necessary. Any doctor whose primary concern is charging you as much money as possible for additional surgeries that you don't need is not for you!

Choosing the Right Doctor

If you've followed all of the suggestions in this chapter and you're still having a difficult time deciding on the right doctor for you, take the following quiz to help you make your final decision.

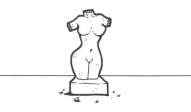

Go Figure!

You will usually be required to pay the full cost of your surgery before you undergo a cosmetic procedure.

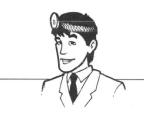

The Doctors Are In

It's also worth checking with your insurance company to find out whether it will cover the cost of any medical expenses related to problems arising from your cosmetic procedure. Some insurance companies will cover these costs, but many will not.

Choosing the Right Doctor Quiz

Is your doctor board certified by the American Board of Plastic Surgery or a member of the American Board of Plastic and Reconstructive Surgeons?
Yes____   No____

Has your doctor performed numerous surgeries like the one you want performed?
Yes____   No____

continues

continued

Has your doctor willingly explained all of the steps and risks involved in your surgery?

Yes____   No____

Is your doctor's operating room fully equipped to handle any life-threatening emergency or any other medical crisis?

Yes____   No____

Will your doctor perform the entire operation?

Yes____   No____

Do you feel comfortable with your doctor's policy about revision surgery?

Yes____   No____

Is your doctor offering your procedure at a price you can afford?

Yes____   No____

Will your doctor be available for aftercare and postoperative questions?

Yes____   No____

Now look over your answers. Whatever doctor can say "yes" to the most questions is the doctor for you. But what if there's a tie between two or more doctors you've interviewed? In that case, answer this final question:

Tiebreaker Question: Which doctor do you feel safe with and trust the most to give you the highest quality of care before, during, and after your surgery?

Choose that doctor!

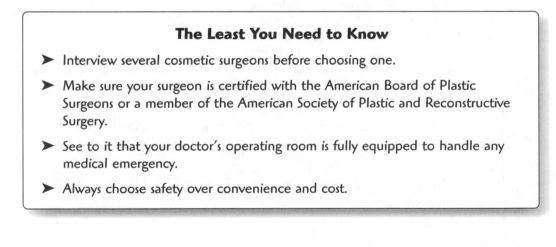

The Least You Need to Know

➤ Interview several cosmetic surgeons before choosing one.

➤ Make sure your surgeon is certified with the American Board of Plastic Surgeons or a member of the American Society of Plastic and Reconstructive Surgery.

➤ See to it that your doctor's operating room is fully equipped to handle any medical emergency.

➤ Always choose safety over convenience and cost.

Part 2

Heavenly Heads and Necks

You've created your own definition of beauty or adopted our definition. You've learned the difference between beauty and cosmetic improvement and your expectations for the results of your surgery or procedure are realistic. You've even decided that you are a candidate for cosmetic improvement, and feel confident that you can choose a board-certified plastic surgeon who is right for you. Now what? Do you think you are ready to make a cosmetic improvement to your face or neck area? After you've read and applied the information in the next section of this book, you will be!

If you are considering making any kind of cosmetic improvement above your shoulders, such as a face-lift, forehead lift, upper- or lower-eyelid surgery, nose surgery, facial-implant surgery, lip enhancement, ear surgery, neck lift, or cosmetic dentistry, then the following chapters will tell you everything you need to know about each operation. After you have become familiar with what to expect before, during, and after each surgery, you can then decide if you would like to proceed with the procedure.

Remember, a fully informed decision is usually the safest decision to make!

Chapter 5

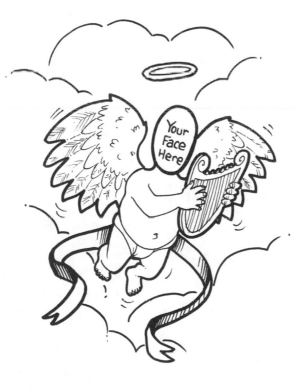

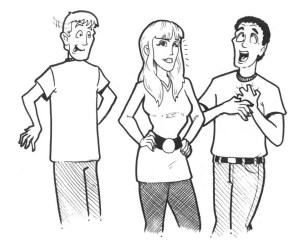

Turning Heads and Breaking Hearts: Face-Lifts

In This Chapter

➤ How face-lifts can turn back the clock

➤ Adding a neck-lift on for good measure

➤ Understanding what face-lifts can't fix

➤ Recovering from your face-lift

Face-lifts are one of the most common cosmetic procedures performed in the field of plastic surgery today. Not only are they common, they can also have the most profound effect on your appearance. For those of you who want to look younger and are approaching the big 4-0, this procedure may be the solution for you if you want to conceal your age and restore your youthful appearance. It can also be the answer for those of you who want to look your age, only better.

Face-lifts (as well as other cosmetic surgeries) can either rejuvenate your youthful appearance or make necessary feature changes to your face that give you a new and improved look without necessarily disguising your age. This chapter will address both rejuvenation techniques and feature changes, because we realize that some of you want to look the same as you did when you were younger and some of you want to look your age, only better!

Your Face and Aging

A youthful facial has clean lines, thick skin that is well-supported by the desirable positioning of the underlying muscles, full lip and mouth areas and full central cheeks. With age, all of these characteristics begin to change: Skin gets thinner, lips, mouths, and cheeks begin to lose their natural fattiness and look hollowed out or thin, and wrinkles begin to form.

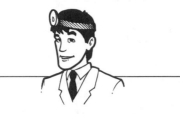

The Doctors Are In

Youth lasts from 18 to 25, when some of the soft buccal fat pads (these are the fat pads in your cheeks that you are born with) start to absorb or slip. Don't hold a surgeon to a higher standard than the material he is working with. When fat is being moved or transplanted, it has a finite life that is unable to be determined. (Nevertheless, it seems to last a long time!)

You can start rejuvenating your face when you first start seeing signs of fraying. When a face first frays,

➤ lips may thin or curve less.

➤ naso-labial folds (the lines that travel from the outside of your nostrils to the corners of your lips) deepen.

➤ cheeks sag.

The "Fix It as You Need It" Approach

Today everyone agrees that early correction, on a "fix it as you need it" basis, is the best approach for most people and provides the longest-lasting results.

Fat Transplants

Face fray is due to loss of face fat, which is commonly caused by weight fluctuation, fatigue, and lack of sleep. One of the best early-intervention techniques is to fill these early signs of face fray with your own fat.

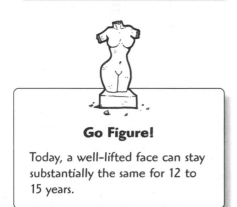

Go Figure!

Today, a well-lifted face can stay substantially the same for 12 to 15 years.

The fat lost in the cheeks and naso-labial folds can be restored with stable fat, which is usually procured from your own hips and inner thighs. Stomach fat fluctuates and is less stable than hip and thigh fat and is easily lost with diet, so if you lose weight and your fat transplants were made from your stomach fat, your transplants may shrink very quickly. But because thigh and hip fat is so much more stable, you can lose weight and will still stand a good chance of keeping your fat transplants if the fat is procured from those areas.

Fat transplants, like skin treatments and hair coloring, require maintenance. If you don't maintain your transplants, you will lose the effect over time.

It's just a fact: There are some cosmetic surgeries that require follow-up treatments. Keep in mind, you aren't stainless steel: You might have to do this from time to time. Nothing is permanent.

Face-Lifts

While there are things that you can do to help re-duce the signs of aging, at some point it's time to face reality and realize that you've reached a level of change that would benefit from a full-blown face-lift. It is best to treat faces and necks early so that less surgery will need to be performed. Typically, you are a good candidate for a face-lift if you have the following characteristics:

➤ Sagging cheeks

➤ Heavy naso-labial fold (the fold of skin from the nostrils to the mouth that develops with age)

➤ Jowls along the jawline

Cosmetic surgeons improve the appearance of your face by removing extra skin on your face which has lost its elasticity over the years and by tighten-ing the tissue under your skin.

Taking Your Neck with You When You Go

Surgeons typically perform neck-lifts along with face-lifts because generally if you need a face-lift, you also need a neck lift. Neck lifts can typically correct double chins, and the prominent bands (called platysmal bands) on your neck. Doctors remedy these problems by removing excess skin, tightening the muscle, and removing excess fat from the neck.

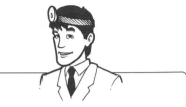

The Doctors Are In

The kind of look that is aesthet-ically desirable will probably always be debated and will cer-tainly change over time. Some surgeons and patients agree on an overcorrected rather than a subtle look. Our professional opinion is that surgery should be undetectable and imitate youth: If there is a flaw, it should be a natural flaw (slight undercorrec-tion) rather than a surgical arti-fact (overcorrection). You'll want to look more natural instead of too pulled.

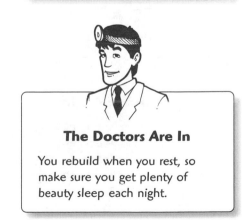

The Doctors Are In

You rebuild when you rest, so make sure you get plenty of beauty sleep each night.

Here's a face and neck before and after a face-lift and neck-lift. Note that the nasolabial folds are corrected, the jowls are removed and the jaw has better definition, and the platysmal bands are reduced.

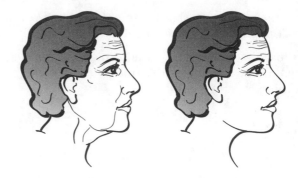

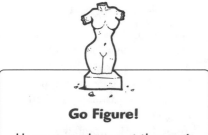

Go Figure!

Hormone-replacement therapy is a less intrusive technique that might be able to help prevent early signs of aging. Ask your doctor for more details about hormone-replacement therapy and find out if it is right for you!

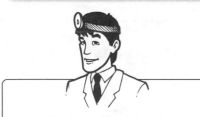

The Doctors Are In

Someone who undergoes planned maintenance of cosmetic procedures is very different than someone who has an addiction to surgery—that is, someone who has too much surgery performed as a way of dealing with life and mortality.

Foreheads and Eyes Alert!

It's important to note that face and neck lifts do not correct wrinkles and lines around the eyes. To improve the appearance of the eyes and forehead you would probably need eyelid surgery (see Chapter 7, "Raising Eye Brows: Eyelid Surgery), a chemical peel (see Chapter 24, "Deep Facials: Chemical Peels and Laser Resurfacing"), and/or a forehead lift (see Chapter 6, "Smoothing Out Your Forehead"). It's common for patients to have all these procedures performed in order for their face to look the same age all over.

The Face-Lift Procedure

Face-lifts require a cosmetic surgeon who is skilled and has a good aesthetic judgment in order to achieve good results. Typically, the surgeon makes an incision that begins above the ear and goes into the ear so that the scar is less detectable, then it goes back behind into the crease of the ear and into the hairline. Another incision will be made under the chin. The scars generally heal well and are well-hidden after one to three months. The exception is the scar behind the ear, which might be visible but can be covered with make-up or your hairstyle.

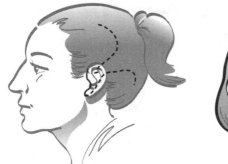

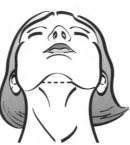

The incisions for a typical face-lift. The scars will be difficult to detect if they heal well. Poor healing usually responds well to scar revision.

Face-Lift Alternatives

We've already discussed some of the alternatives to a full-blown face-lift in this chapter, and you'll be glad to know that some face-lifts can even be postponed or avoided with fat transplants (check out Chapter 25, "Get the Skin You Want Now! Soft-Tissue Augmentation," for more information about this rejuvenating alternative). Peeling and liposculpture of both the neck and perhaps the eyes could also be performed instead of a face-lift in some instances (see Chapter 24). All of these alternative procedures will likely require maintenance to keep the results.

Not Necessarily Younger, but Better

A face-lift can't create features that you didn't already have when you were younger. When your cosmetic goal is more than just looking younger, but to also look prettier or more handsome, then look into cheek and chin implants (see Chapter 9, "Face Your Facial-Implant Options") or a nose job

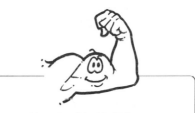

Better Definition

You might have heard of a procedure called an endoscopic face-lift, which is performed through small incisions in the face using an instrument called an endoscope. The procedure is desirable because it requires far fewer incisions, but it isn't very effective if you have excess skin (which most people who want to have a face-lift have) because no skin can be removed during this kind of a procedure. Not all surgeons embrace this technique.

(see Chapter 8, "Follow Your Nose! Nose Jobs"). These are common alterations that many people consider when they want to improve their appearance.

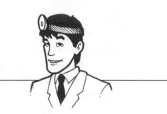

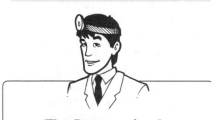

Facing Your Face-Lift Recovery

The old rules are still true: The first week you rest. Your head is elevated and you stay on your back. Since a face-lift is a major surgery that requires your body to work overtime to heal, you will probably be exceptionally tired. You can also anticipate losing some weight due to loss of appetite, increased metabolism of healing, and other common side effects that most people experience after surgery. Keep in mind that the more you sleep, the faster you will heal.

The second week of your recovery, you might be bored and want to get out of the house, but you will still not be ready for public presentation and will need to rest in order to maintain an uncomplicated recovery period. However, if your surgery is not a secret, you can be back to work or fly home after 12 to 14 days—but not any sooner than that.

For the surgery to be a complete secret, you'll need three to four weeks to adequately heal in order to conceal most signs of surgery. Most people are back to work in two weeks, but no one will be making a movie before the third week. So don't expect to look like a movie star a few weeks after your surgery, unless you came in looking like one. Remember, you will have healed adequately enough to conceal the signs of your surgery, but you will still be healing and your recovery period may take several months. The contour and shape of your face will still be changing.

The more you sleep, the faster you will heal. It is better not to chew the first week after surgery. You won't want to move your jaw much at all, since this would stretch your face and it could cause swelling or weakening of the muscles or your stitches to come undone. Instead, write notes to those you need to converse with. Maintain a high-protein, vitamin-filled, preservative-free liquid diet so you will receive the proper nutrition you need during your recovery without compromising your healing process. Avoid any exertion that might induce swelling. Also, keep in mind that you cannot have a face-lift and fly off to a vacation spot to heal. You should be near your doctor in case any complications arise.

A Face-Lift Checklist

Before you have your face-lift, use this list to determine if you are really ready for surgery. Make sure that you know and feel comfortable with all the answers to the following questions:

1. Is the doctor trained in cosmetic surgery?
   Yes_____ No_____

2. Is the anesthesiologist trained in anesthesia?
   Yes_____ No_____

3. Can you continue to take your prescription medications or over-the-counter treatments before your surgery?
   Yes_____ No_____

4. Where will the incisions be placed?
   Yes_____ No_____

5. How is your hairline affected?
   Yes_____ No_____

6. Will your earlobes be the same?
   Yes_____ No_____

7. How tight do you want your face to look? What compromises will I have to make since this is only repair, not rejuvenation?
   Yes_____ No_____

8. Rather than cosmetic surgery, what might you accomplish through diet, hormones, exercise, and supplements?
   Yes_____ No_____

Remember, the doctor is not a magician. He can repair and improve but he cannot make you young. Recent advances in supplements, vitamins, exercise, hormones, and hormonal precursors might make a big difference in how well you age.

Facing the Money Facts

The fees for face-lift procedures are usually all-inclusive and are not itemized. Regional variation in costs is not as common as it once was, but experience and training is often factored into the price.

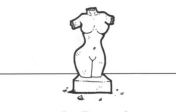

Go Figure!

More and more men are having face-lift surgery. They usually don't want or need to look as tight as women, but their incisions need to be just as hidden!

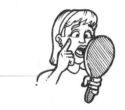

Wrinkle Ahead!

When you feel your face is beginning to fray, fix it! But if you can't see freying in a photograph, don't bother to operate on it.

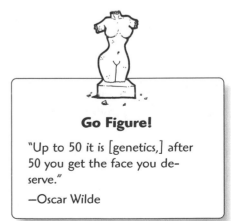

Go Figure!

"Up to 50 it is [genetics,] after 50 you get the face you deserve."

—Oscar Wilde

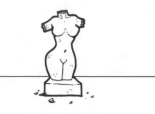

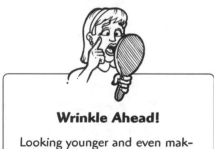

Go Figure!

Sometimes with the early signs of aging, the restoration of the soft tissue with fat transplants is sufficient enough to put off more extensive surgery for a number of years.

Wrinkle Ahead!

Looking younger and even making some minor feature changes are OK, but we recommend that you don't have so much surgery performed at one time that no one will recognize you.

A doctor generally does factor certain costs into the price when a global fee is presented.

Anesthesia

Anesthesia for a face-lift usually costs $200–$250 an hour (plus a start-up charge). Because they typically charge an hourly rate, you'll save money with a faster, more experienced surgeon. Anesthesia for a face-lift (including a neck-lift) can cost $1,000 because the anesthesiologist will stay with you before and after the surgery. Recovery care is important and ethically should be provided.

Operating Room Costs

Surgeons typically charge around $1,500 to cover the cost of maintaining a certified operating room, sterilization techniques, and generators (which are necessary in case the electricity goes out during a procedure). Hospitals might charge $500 an hour for care during surgery, and extra for recovery care. The same care in an outpatient facility of a hospital could be $3,000–$3,500. The outpatient center provided by the surgeon is a bargain.

The Check, Please ...

All-inclusive fees for face-lifts vary between $7,000 and $10,000, depending on if the procedure has been done before and how much has to be done. The neck-lift can be included with the face-lift if it is needed.

So now that you know what you can do to achieve a more youthful face and neck, don't wait until everything falls apart to fix it; it might be almost too late to enjoy the cosmetic changes or too late to have an impact on your life. Remember, as soon as anything begins to fray, fix it!

The Least You Need to Know

➤ Consider having a face-lift and neck lift if you have heavy naso-labial folds, jowls, or a double chin.

➤ Rejuvenating early signs of aging as they appear can delay a full-blown face-lift for several years.

➤ Remember that a face-lift cannot correct crows feet or forehead lines.

➤ Allow yourself a full two weeks of recovery time after your procedure.

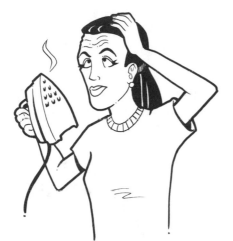

Smoothing Out Your Forehead

In This Chapter

➤ Identifying signs of aging and what you can do about them

➤ Looking at nonsurgical options for smoothing out your forehead

➤ Considering three ways to lift your forehead

➤ How to determine if a forehead lift is right for you

The skin of a young person's forehead is typically thick and fairly smooth, and is framed by a full head of hair. But with age, people's foreheads often begin to accumulate lines and skin droops, causing them to look tired, angry, or just plain old! In this chapter we'll show you what you can do to recapture your forehead of youth—and maybe even improve upon it!

By the time you finish reading this chapter, you'll know what you can do to postpone the signs of aging on your forehead and, once they appear, what you can do to reduce them.

Your Forehead and Aging

Time, the sun, your lifestyle, and gravity all take their toll on your forehead. The most common forehead characteristics that people like to have improved upon or removed altogether are:

➤ Horizontal wrinkles—ranging from slight to crevice-like—creasing the brow and causing people to look older or tired.

➤ Permanent scowl lines above the nose and between the brows that give people a perpetually angry or irritated look.

➤ Droopy eyebrows that fall below their original position.

➤ Folds of skin at the outside corner of each eye (called lateral hoods) that contribute to your looking old and tired.

Signs of aging on the forehead and the same forehead after a forehead lift procedure. Note that the horizontal creases, scowl lines, droopy eyebrows, and lateral hoods have all been improved.

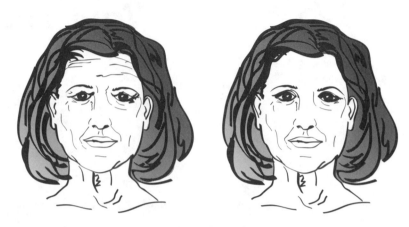

If you have any or all of these characteristics, there's good news: they can be improved upon or possibly even eliminated altogether! In the next few sections of this chapter we will describe both nonsurgical and surgical procedures available to give you back the forehead of your youth.

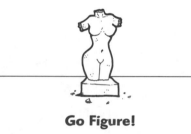

Go Figure!

Ever take a good, long look at someone's forehead? If the answer is "no," then you're like most people. That's because we really don't pay attention to foreheads unless something is wrong with them.

Nonsurgical Forehead Improvements

Surgery isn't the only solution available for reducing signs of aging such as skin drooping and lines, and you should consider these before you agree to any cosmetic surgery:

➤ **Scrubs and peels.** Light lines that develop early in the aging process can be reduced with self-peeling products and scrubs.

➤ **Chemical peels.** Superficial and medium chemical peels can improve the tone of the skin as well as reduce the appearance of lines on the forehead caused by sun damage and aging. See Chapter 24, "Deep Facials: Chemical Peels and Laser Resurfacing," for more information.

➤ **Fat transplants.** Fat transplanted from your own body can also be used to smooth and thicken a forehead at almost any age. Chapter 25, "Get the Skin You Want Now! Soft-Tissue Augmentation," has more information on fat transplants.

➤ **Botox.** If you have lines, Botox can cause temporary paralysis of the muscles in the forehead and thus smooth out the lines (also discussed in Chapter 25). When you paralyze muscles, they atrophy and get thin. Long-term use will thin these muscles and can contribute to an altered look.

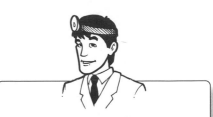

The Doctors Are In

If you wear sunglasses when you're out in the sun and maintain the correct prescription in your eyeglasses, you stand a good chance of keeping your forehead looking great for a long time to come!

When Surgery Is the Best Way

A forehead lift is just that: Your skin and muscle are "lifted" or shifted upward, which raises your brows and lateral hoods and "unwrinkles" your horizontal wrinkles. There are three different ways that foreheads are typically raised, and we'll discuss each of them in this section.

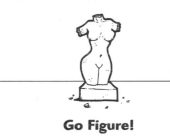

Go Figure!

Botox, which paralyzes muscles and thus reduces the appearance of lines, demonstrates that if you don't move your forehead, it smooths out!

Endoscopic Lift

The endoscopic forehead lift is the procedure of choice for many people because it doesn't require the long incisions that the other two kinds of procedures do. During an endoscopic forehead lift, your cosmetic surgeon will make four-six short vertical incisions on your head behind your hairline, and the skin of your forehead is pulled up and held in place with temporary screws.

The incision marks for the endoscopic lift. The success rate for this surgery is undetermined and recurrence does happen. The scars are supposed to be hidden in the hairline but this is not always the case.

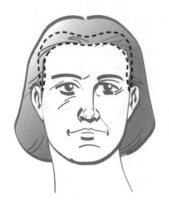

The endoscopic procedure isn't the right procedure for everyone, as it isn't as capable of removing severe horizontal wrinkles and scowl lines as the forehead lifts that involve long scars. The procedure also pulls up your hairline at the same time that it pulls up your forehead, so if you already have a high forehead, this procedure probably isn't for you.

The Coronal Lift

During a coronal lift procedure your cosmetic surgeon will create a single or pair of incisions at the top of your head that extends from ear to ear, and will pull the skin and muscle back and there will be no excess skin. Hair will need to be removed and skin will be reattached at incision site. When the scar is in the hairline it can still be seen and sometimes the scar can spread, which causes the appearance of hair loss.

There are disadvantages to the coronal lift, which include:

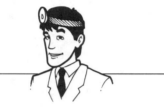

The Doctors Are In

Many cosmetic surgeons use peeling as a way to shrink and smooth forehead skin without cutting it. No nerves are damaged in the process and there is minimal risk of scars developing. It should be considered as an alternative to a forehead lift if you have mild signs of aging.

➤ Scalp numbness will likely be experienced for several months following surgery and can even be permanent.

➤ The hairline will be raised, so people with high foreheads should avoid this procedure.

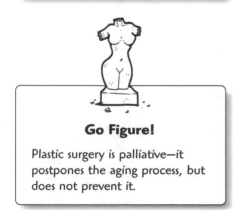

Go Figure!

Plastic surgery is palliative—it postpones the aging process, but does not prevent it.

72

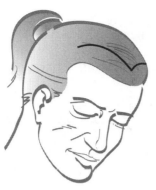

Incision line for a coronal lift, note that the incision runs across the top of the head but behind the hairline.

Subcutaneous Lift

The subcutaneous lift involves your surgeon making an incision line directly under your hairline and pulling the skin up. The excess skin is then removed, and the skin is reattached at the incision line. Because the incision is placed just below the hairline, the hairline itself is not raised, making this an ideal procedure for people with high foreheads who don't wish to have them go any higher. This procedure also avoids the numbing that is involved with a coronal lift.

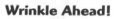

Wrinkle Ahead!

Sometimes people think they need their eyebrows raised with a forehead lift when what they really need is upper eyelid surgery to reduce excess skin. Make sure you discuss your goals with your cosmetic surgeon so she or he knows what characteristics you want corrected.

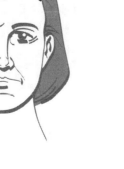

Incision line for a subcutaneous lift. The scar will be visible if you don't wear your hair with bangs to cover it.

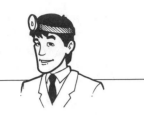

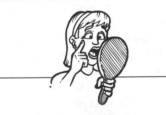

The major drawback to a subcutaneous lift is the scar, which will be visible when the hair is pulled back. Consequently, this procedure isn't recommended for people who will want to wear their hair in a style that is pulled off of their forehead.

What a Forehead Lift Can't Correct

Although forehead lifts can have a dramatic affect on your appearance, giving you a tighter look, they are not effective for some problems, for which you'll need to address through other solutions. These include:

➤ Crows feet. Consider having Botox injections or laser or chemical resurfacing (see Chapter 25 for more on Botox, and Chapter 24 for information on skin resurfacing).

➤ Excess eyelid skin. Check out Chapter 7, "Raising Eyebrows: Eyelid Surgery" for how these can be improved.

➤ Poor skin tone. Consider having a chemical or laser peel, as discussed in Chapter 24.

Is All This for You?

You may be wondering if you are the ideal candidate for a forehead lift. It is not a good place to take risks you're not willing to accept. Lifted foreheads respond best if you have a low forehead and thick black hair. Any change you make needs to suit both your features and how you view yourself.

Before you decide that a forehead lift is what you need, consult with your physician and review our criteria in the next section to make sure that you are indeed a good candidate for this surgery. You won't want to make a mistake with your face—it's the only one you'll ever have!

Do You Have the Right Characteristics for a Forehead Lift?

We can't emphasize enough that the desire alone for cosmetic surgery does not mean that forehead-lift surgery (or any other kind of surgery, for that matter) should be performed on you. If you do not take the time to consider a few simple facts about your appearance, you may end up disliking your results:

➤ **Drastically low-browed, dark-haired people.** The ideal candidate is someone who has thick black hair and a drastically low, wrinkled brow. The results of surgery on people with these characteristics are dramatic because the patient not only gets the hair out of his or her eyes, but gets a smooth forehead at the same time. Interestingly, people with these characteristics also tend to have thick skin, which improves in appearance when stretched. There aren't a lot of people who fit these criteria, but patients who have them see very great improvement in their appearance from forehead-lift surgery.

➤ **Short foreheads.** If your forehead is short, but not as drastically short as described above, you still can benefit from this surgery.

When a Forehead Lift Might Not Be Right for You

So now you know which features respond best to a forehead lift procedure, how about those features that might not be well-suited to the surgery? Read on!

➤ **Thin hair.** Don't have a forehead lift if you have thin hair. When your doctor makes an incision in the hair, the site behind the incision is stretched and thins the hair. When your hair is coarse and thick, it doesn't seem to be affected by this

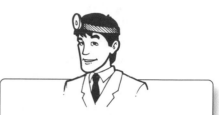

The Doctors Are In

There is a present-day fad to lift the eyebrows higher than they ever were originally and to move the hairline back no matter how high your forehead is. This makes a person look like a surgical product of a certain time, and will date him or her as much as a chignon would were it affected today.

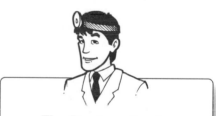

The Doctors Are In

People are divided on the topic of how "operated on" someone should look and how high an eyebrow should be. In the 1980s it was vogue to undergo procedures that didn't necessarily hide the fact that cosmetic surgery was performed. We must credit comedy writer Beth Lapidis with her comment that plastic surgery in the '80s was much like a math problem: "Show your work."

process. But with less hardy hair, the change in the tensions is reflected in further decreased hair density.

➤ **Blond hair.** People with blond hair have the greatest number of hairs per square inch, but because blond hair is pale, it doesn't always cover large scars well. When you stretch the scalp (which happens during forehead lifts), the hair appears thinner than ever, making the scar visible. Even if the scar is well behind the hairline, people with blond hair will likely still have to conceal it. Furthermore, people with blond hair usually have normal or high foreheads, which would be exaggerated in length by the advancement or stretching of the forehead.

➤ **High eyebrows.** If you have high brows, you already face the possibility of people thinking that you've had a face-or forehead lift—even without moving your features to places they have never been before.

➤ **High forehead.** If you already have a high forehead, then a forehead lift will increase the height of your forehead, giving you an undesirable result.

Someone with an average size forehead and eyebrows that fall in a normal position (left) and the possible side effects if the brows and hairline are raised too high during a forehead lift. These problems are almost impossible to correct.

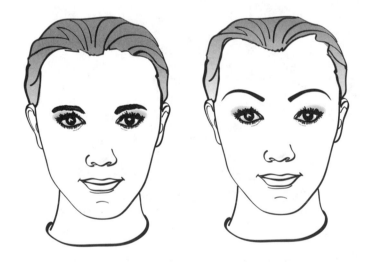

If you have characteristics that will prevent you from having desirable results, consider smoothing your forehead with chemical peels or other soft-tissue augmentation procedures. They are relatively safe and fast-healing when performed by experienced hands.

The Cost of Your New Forehead

Forehead lifts typically cost around $5,000, including anesthesia and operating room costs.

Before Your Surgery: Evening Out the Rough Spots

Preparation for forehead-lift surgery is simple and easy. Here are some helpful preoperative hints that we think you can benefit from before your surgery. These tips will help you to even out the rough spots and get you in optimum condition for your operation!

➤ **Don't change shampoos.** Now isn't the time to change shampoos. Your hair may be in shock after surgery and you won't want it to have to adjust to a new shampoo. Make it easy on your hair by using your regular shampoo. Also, use plenty of conditioner. Your hair will need the extra help.

➤ **If you color your hair, do it before surgery.** You won't be able to color your hair for three weeks after surgery. Get a color crayon if you will have to go out in public. Don't change colors before surgery, because it can weaken your hair, making it more prone to damage during the procedure.

➤ **No new short hairstyles.** You will want to leave that for later. Your surgery will already alter your appearance. You will want to estimate whether or not you like your results after your surgery. Additionally altering your appearance with a new hairstyle may skew your view of your surgical results. You might decide that you dislike the results of your surgery, when it is actually your new hairstyle that is unbecoming. Avoid skewing your view and save experimenting with a new, shorter hairstyle later.

➤ **Take vitamins.** Since surgery can be a shock to the hair, take vitamins, gelatin, and proteins for a long period before the planned surgery. You want to maintain good nutrition but not gain weight. Remember to count the calories.

➤ **Take Arnica.** Arnica, and herbal supplement, has been shown to be effective in controlling and reducing bruising. Started well before surgery (weeks), it should be continued through the postoperative period and weeks afterward until you are certain there is no risk of further bruising.

If you follow these simple suggestions, we promise that you'll feel better sooner!

Smoothing It Over

Now that we've evened out the rough spots of the preoperative phase of your forehead surgery, allow us to smooth over the recuperation phase of your operation. Here are a few short and simple tips to follow:

➤ Don't overtreat your hair with brushing or treatments. You can spread your scar.

➤ Keep the site dry unless it has been sealed with a cyanoacrylate glue, otherwise complications could occur!

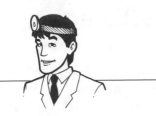

The Doctors Are In

Remember that surgical procedures have periods of being in fashion, just as certain looks do. You will most likely outlive any fashion, so make sure you choose a procedure you can live with for a lifetime.

➤ If you must go out, the site may be covered with a scarf, but not makeup. Putting makeup on the site is not the problem, but you cannot get it off completely without some risk to the surgery or incision site.

➤ If your doctor allows you to wash your hair, use your regular shampoo. Use your regular conditioner, too, because the hair is particularly dry and unmanageable after surgery due to a lack of oils in the scalp from this experience.

These helpful hints will help to ensure a safe and speedy recovery period for you!

Now that you know what procedures are available and have a good sense of whether you are an appropriate candidate for any of them, we encourage you to make an appointment for a consult with your doctor!

The Least You Need to Know

➤ Recognize the signs of aging on your face that can be improved through cosmetic surgery.

➤ Be sure to consider nonsurgical options for correcting your problem before going under the knife.

➤ Discuss the three forehead procedures with your cosmetic surgeon to determine which one, if any, is most appropriate for you.

➤ Don't expect a forehead lift to correct crows feet or excess eyelid skin.

Chapter 7

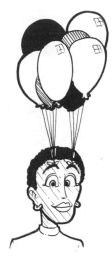

Raising Eyebrows: Eyelid Surgery

In This Chapter

➤ Why people have eyelid surgery

➤ Taking a look at different kinds of eyelid procedures

➤ What you can expect to pay for your eyelid surgery

➤ How to prepare for surgery

➤ Taking care of yourself after your procedure

Poets, songwriters, and novelists have all waxed poetic about eyes. Our eyes are not only our windows onto the world, they are also other people's windows into us. People look us in the eye when they talk to us, and it is often our eyes that reveal what we are really feeling and thinking. It only makes sense, then, that we want our eyes to be as attractive as they can be.

Eyelid surgery is one of the most common cosmetic surgeries performed today. Thousands of eyelid surgeries are performed each year in the United States alone, and most people who have the procedure are happy with the results. It can make anyone look younger, and the results last for a very long time—often a lifetime. Read on to find out all about eyelid surgery and if it's right for you.

Why Operate on the Eyes?

As with most cosmetic procedures, people have many different reasons for choosing to have their eyes operated on. Most people undergo eyelid surgery in order to give themselves a younger, well-rested, and less angry appearance. Sometimes, though, people might already have a youthful appearance but want to change the shape of their eye.

Opening Your Eyes to a More Youthful Appearance

Eyelid surgery can decrease signs of aging and make you look much younger and more energetic. The following problems can be corrected or minimized with eyelid surgery:

➤ **Drooping upper eyelids.** Ideal eyelids cover the very edge of the bottom of the *iris* (for lower eyelids) and top of the iris (for upper eyelids). If your upper eyelids are droopy, they will cover more of the iris and, if too low, can interfere with your ability to see, although, this is rare. Droopy upper eyelids often cause people to look fatigued.

➤ **Drooping lower eyelids.** If your lower eyelids are droopy, then the whites of your eyes below your iris will be exposed. Droopy lower eyelids can cause dry eyes and excessively droopy lower eyelids look unnatural.

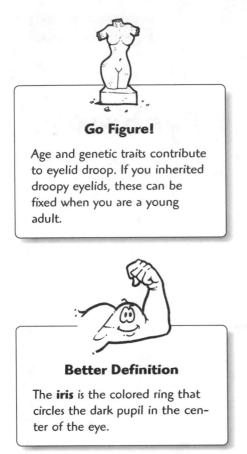

Go Figure!

Age and genetic traits contribute to eyelid droop. If you inherited droopy eyelids, these can be fixed when you are a young adult.

Better Definition

The **iris** is the colored ring that circles the dark pupil in the center of the eye.

This upper and lower eyelids of this eye rest in a normal position right at the edge of the iris.

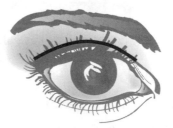

➤ **Puffy eyelids.** Protruding or puffy eyelids are caused by excess fat surrounding the eye. Weight loss does not reduce the puffiness, but the fat can be reduced during surgery. The removal of all the fat will give a "hollow" look that is unfavorable.

➤ **Excess eyelid skin.** If you can pinch excess skin on your upper eyelids when they are closed, then you probably have excess eyelid skin, which contributes to a tired or old-looking appearance.

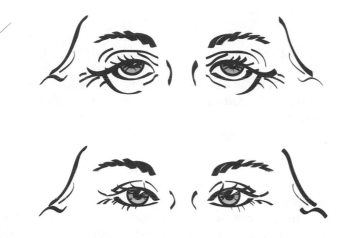

Here's an illustration of what eyelid surgery can improve. The patient had droopy lower and upper lids, excess skin, and puffy lids. The eyes are greatly improved and look much younger after surgery.

Changing the Shape of Your Eyes

Sometimes we just don't like the shape of our eyes. People of Asian descent, for example, have been changing their almond-shaped eyes to a rounder, more Eurasian-looking eye for several years via a technique called "double-eyelid surgery." This procedure produces the kind of eye someone might have been born with if they had a parent or grandparent from another culture, and it is a natural-looking result. As we've said before, a natural-looking result is a great result! No one should end up looking like a surgical product.

While eyelid surgery can be very effective for changing the shape of eyes, particularly giving people with Asian eyes a more Eurasian appearance, it is important to point out that cosmetic surgery cannot make your eyes bigger.

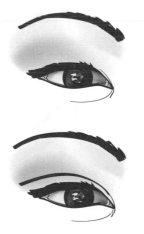

An Asian-looking eyelid.

Asian eyelid after double-eyelid surgery.

Eyelid Procedures

Eyelid surgery is a catchall phrase that includes a few different procedures. Cosmetic surgeons can perform surgery on the upper eyelid and the lower eyelid, and they can also extract excess fat from around the eyes in order to cosmetically enhance the eyes. The type of procedure appropriate for you depends on your eyes and should be discussed with your cosmetic surgeon.

Upper Eyelid Surgery

Upper eyelid surgery is performed to trim away excess skin, to remove excess fat from under the eyelid if it is necessary, and to correct droopy upper eyelids. Your cosmetic surgeon will create an incision in the upper eyelid, making sure that the scar will follow the natural crease of your eyelid and thus be very difficult to detect when healed. Your doctor would make the same incision during double eyelid surgery to create a fold in Asian eyes.

The incisions for upper eyelid surgery will be difficult to detect when the scars heal.

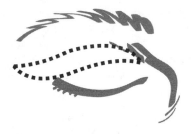

Lower Eyelid Surgery

The incision for lower eyelid surgery is usually placed just under the eyelashes and will ideally be hard to find if all heals well because it follows the natural wrinkles in under your eyes. Your doctor will be able to extract excess fat and skin through this incision.

The incisions for lower eyelid surgery will be hard to find if the scars heal well.

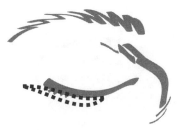

The Eyelid and Midface-Lift Combo

If you need it, you might be able to get a midface-lift (also called a cheek lift) when you have your lower lids done. It is one way to make the area around your eyes look younger when you have eyelid surgery performed.

A midface-lift is not related to lower-lid surgery except that it can be performed through an undetectable incision inside of the eye. This area will already have to have incisions made into it to perform a lower-lid surgery anyway, so it makes sense to have a midface-lift performed (if you need one) at the same time. A midface-lift involves lifting the muscle around the cheek to reduce the appearance of the heavy folds (naso-labial folds) between your lower lids and mouth, and the procedure only creates muscle suspension for the midface. When you are ready to have your lower eyelid surgery performed, ask your doctor whether or not he or she would also recommend a midface-lift. If this is done, it needs to be done conservatively—remember that a little bit of surgery goes a long way, and it's important not to have your surgeon "over correct" your condition.

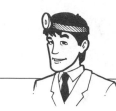

The Doctors Are In

In some cases when you might think your eyes need cosmetic surgery, it's other areas of your face that are causing the problem. Instead of eyelid surgery, you might need to lift the sagging tissue adjacent to the eyes if it is no longer providing support to the eyes.

The Eyelid and Chemical Peel Combo

Some people have eyelid surgery more than once in their lifetime, but there are things you can do to make your first eyelid surgery last longer. If your eyes are peeled at the same time that you have your eyelid surgery, the texture of the skin around your eyes will be smoother and the tightness of this skin will last longer than if you do not have them peeled. Even if you don't peel your eyes when you have eyelid surgery, they can be peeled, usually very effectively, years after your original surgery. Peels usually freshen up the appearance of your eyelid surgery. See Chapter 24, "Deep Facials: Chemical Peels and Laser Resurfacing," for more skin-freshening techniques.

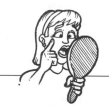

Wrinkle Ahead!

The midface-lift is a fairly new procedure, and it should be approached with caution. Because it moves the muscle in your midface, it can result in a different looking face—not just a *younger-looking* face, but a *different-looking* one. It can also cause a lot of swelling that might not go down for several months.

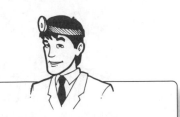

The Doctors Are In

Our recommendation is to be sure that your surgeon does not place incisions all the way along the outside of your lower eyelids during this operation; the scars will show and this kind of incision placement may contribute to too-round eye shape developing later on. Be sure your surgeon is conservative in his or her approach and conserves as much fat as possible so that your eyes do not look too large or hollow.

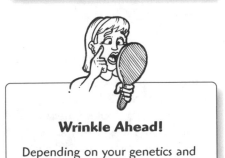

Wrinkle Ahead!

Depending on your genetics and the life you have lived, your eyes may be a bit more difficult than others to freshen up; over a long period of time, drinking, smoking, and sun tanning can have a wearing effect on that area of the body.

Be Careful About What You Ask For ...

For some doctors and patients alike, eyelid surgery is a catchall for fixing features that might better benefit from another type of cosmetic surgery, or it is used for fixing a prior cosmetic operation that caused a patient's eyes to become too round. Sometimes a fat transplant will raise a sagging brow or fill a hollow eyelid. Or someone may want eyelid surgery to correct upper- or lower-lid skin that has a crepe paper-like texture to it when what he or she really needs is a peel to smooth out the texture.

Keep these facts in mind and be sure that what you want to correct or enhance about your eyelids really requires surgery instead of a minor cosmetic procedure.

The Incredible Shrinking Eye Syndrome

If you decide to have your lids surgically enhanced, keep in mind that modern surgery should be fat-sparing at both the upper and lower lid. If your doctor removes too much upper-lid fat, it will make your eyes look too hollow; if he or she removes too much lower-lid fat, it will make your lower lids get smaller over time because they tend to sink back into the eye socket. When fat is left behind, there is a chance that more fat will return, but this is much more desirable than what we call "the incredible shrinking eye syndrome."

Eyes that shrink from surgery can yield an older appearance—exactly what most of us hope to avoid by having cosmetic surgery. The next time you see someone over 60, notice how as a natural part of the aging process they tend to have little eyes from the loss of the fat pads around their eyes. This is what you might end up looking like if you or your doctor suggests that too much fat be removed from around your eyes during eyelid surgery. There are other ways of making you look younger.

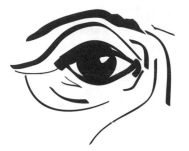

An eye that has had too much fat removed. The only way to insure against having too much fat removed during eyelid surgery is to use a skilled and experienced surgeon.

Raising Eyebrows

If all of this information has caused you to raise an eyebrow and wonder if you are a candidate for this surgery, then consider making an appointment for an initial consult with a cosmetic surgeon.

But before you decide to see your doctor, consider the following facts. It is always a good idea to be well-informed about all options involved in any surgery you are contemplating.

When in Doubt, Cut It Out!

If you have extra upper- or lower-lid skin, it can be removed. Some people incorrectly believe that they must be a certain age to have extra skin removed because age naturally causes this to happen for many people. While it is true that extra upper- and lower-lid skin often develops with age, it is also true that some people are genetically predisposed to have extra skin above or below their eyes naturally. If you have doubts about the extra skin that is sagging or drooping above or below your eyes, talk to your cosmetic surgeon about having it surgically removed—no matter how old or young you are.

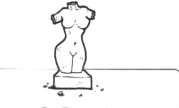

Go Figure!

Betcha didn't know people of different ethnicities have different kinds of fat! There is a basic difference in the type of fat in most Asian eyes compared to Western or European eyes. Asian fat is distributed in little droplets, while Western fat is in large globules. There are about four globules in the Western lower lid and about three in the upper. However, there are no absolutes: Variations and combinations of this fat distribution appear irregularly in all races of people.

Stay in Shape!

If you have extra fat, it can be removed at the nose and outside corner of the eye. However, not all of it has to be removed. Remember, you can and should keep some of it so that you do not end up with too hollow of an eye. Also, you might not want

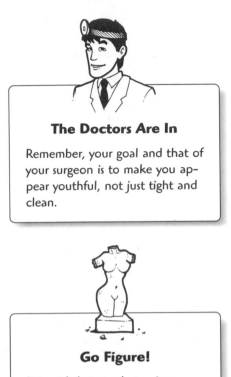

to lose the personal shape of your own eye. Unless you want a feature change, keep the shape of your eye by having only a partial amount of the fat removed at the corners of each eye.

A Stitch in Time Saves Nine

There is no reason to wait beyond the first signs of drooping or puffiness to have eyelid surgery. Once eyes are fixed, they tend to stay fixed. Having this operation performed sooner rather than later will only mean that you will have good results sooner and for a longer period of time than if you waited and had them done later. Eyes generally only need to be done once or twice in a lifetime, and as we mentioned earlier, they can always be refreshed with light peeling on an as-needed basis. There is no need to wait until your upper-lid skin is over your lashes or your lower lids are very puffy to consult with a cosmetic surgeon.

Create a Feature Change

Maybe you do not have heavy, sagging, or puffy eyes, but you would like to change the shape of your eyes. In other words, you would like to create a feature change. In this case, eyelid surgery would be for you, and we recommend that you have it done at your earliest opportunity because the younger you are, the quicker you will heal. In addition, you will be able to enjoy the results sooner and they will stay with you through most if not all of your adult life.

Create an Ethnic Change

If you have almond-shaped eyes due to your genetics and would like a more-rounded appearance, your eyes can be surgically reshaped. For instance, people with Asian backgrounds who have more narrow and almond-shaped eyes can surgically alter them to create a less narrow and more rounded appearance. This ethnic change has been in popular demand over the last decade.

Just a Quick Trim and Lift!

If you have heavy lower lids and heavy skin folds between your lower lids and your mouth (naso-labial folds), the muscles contributing to this can be lifted upward and even trimmed as your lower-lid muscles are controlled through lower eyelid surgery. Some people refer to this as a midface-lift, which we described earlier in this chapter. Take this into account when you have decided that you are a candidate for lower eyelid surgery and decide whether or not a midface-lift is for you.

A Longer Look

If the corners of your eyes naturally droop or tend to droop as a result from a prior surgery, you can have this repaired and even create the slight appearance of a longer and more dramatic eye.

Lift It Up or Cut It Out?

Some people are being told they need their eyebrows raised when they just need their upper eyelid skin surgically trimmed. If your eyebrows were lifted up, it would pull the upper lid of your skin, and if this were performed surgically, it would permanently leave your brows in way too high of a position. This is probably not the natural location of where your brows were at any time in your life, including your youth. So, you are left with the choice of lifting up your eyebrows or having the extra skin on your upper lids surgically cut out in order to regain a more youthful appearance. For the sake of a natural appearance, we say, have the extra skin surgically removed.

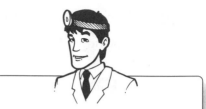

The Doctors Are In

If you have puffy eyes, it makes even more sense to correct it early, because it will stabilize your eye and holds the fullness from sagging or causing the sag from moving forward and causing further drooping. Waiting to have surgery might result in the skin around your eyes stretching, causing you to need more surgery than if you caught it early and had the operation. Remember, a stitch in time saves nine!

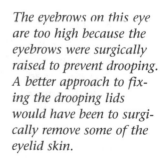

The eyebrows on this eye are too high because the eyebrows were surgically raised to prevent drooping. A better approach to fixing the drooping lids would have been to surgically remove some of the eyelid skin.

Watch for Thinning

Feel the ridge of the forehead above your eyes. It is prominent in men and softer (but still detectable) in women. This is the area that the eyebrow pads and protects, and if it is thinning, it can cause your forehead to droop. This can be controlled with a fat transplant to restore thickness. Watch for thinning and drooping in this area.

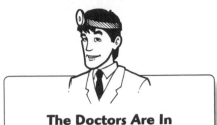

The Doctors Are In

We suggest that you have the least amount of surgery performed in order to get the greatest amount of results. You want to look normal and youthful, not operated on and stretched. Cutting your brows to spite your face isn't going to recapture your youth.

Get the Skinny on Fat

If your upper eyelids are beginning to droop or already drooping but your brows are at the right height, don't fix it upward. Just address the upper-eyelid skin or eyelid fat. You may need to treat one or both.

You Can't Get Bigger Eyes!

Eye surgery does not make your eyes any bigger. Instead, it can give the appearance of larger eyes by trimming away the extra skin that surrounds the upper and/or lower parts of your eyes. It is a myth that eyelid surgery actually increases the eye size.

Your Beauty Checklist

Still confused about what procedure might be most appropriate for your features? We've created a beauty checklist that recaps what we've discussed in this chapter:

➤ If you have extra skin around your eyes, upper and lower eyelid surgery can help. If you are unhappy with the texture of your eyelid skin, eyelid surgery cannot help your condition—you should consider having the skin chemically resurfaced.

➤ Look at your profile. If your forehead is not prominent, you will not get as good of a result with upper-lid surgery as someone who does have a prominent forehead. Those with prominent foreheads have a facial bone structure that support upper-eyelid surgery. The skin tends to drape better on this type of bone structure.

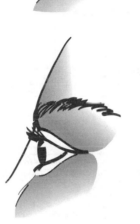

The ideal candidate for upper-eyelid surgery has a prominent forehead.

When the eyes bulge out farther than the forehead, there are folds that cannot be removed. The result of eyelid surgery can be good, but it won't be as good as someone with a more prominent forehead.

➤ If you have smile lines in your naso-labial folds that go from the inner corners of your eyes or outer edges of your nose to the outer edges of your mouth, lower-eyelid surgery will not help. Thickening the skin via skin care (see Chapter 24), having a midface-lift, or utilizing a soft-tissue augmentation technique (see Chapter 25) can help your condition.

➤ If you have extra skin on your upper lids when you look upward, then you are a candidate for upper-eyelid surgery.

➤ If your cheek area is loose, you may eventually need face-lift surgery. Notice the tightness or looseness of your lateral cheekbone area. You may not need this now, but if your eyes lose their good look over the next few years, it may be that your cheeks are getting loose. Repeating eyelid surgery will not solve this problem, but a midface-lift will.

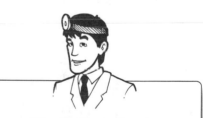

The Doctors Are In

If you wear glasses or contacts, eyelid surgery can change your prescription a little bit because of the change in pressures on the globes of your eyes. Get an eye exam a couple of months after surgery and change your prescription then if needed.

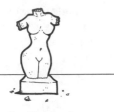

Go Figure!

The more surgery you have done at once, the less the fee is per site because you are already under anesthesia. Also, necessary incisions for your additional operation frequently have already been made because they were needed for your initial operation.

Consider the Cost

People often have another procedure performed when they have eyelid surgery, and with the addition of procedures, the costs will go up.

A global fee for simple eyelid surgery (total cost for both eyes, upper and lower) ranges between $4,500 and $5,500.

A combination of lower-lid surgery and a midface-lift will cost between $3,500 and $4,000.

We hope these facts have helped you to decide whether or not you are a likely candidate for this operation. Remember, catching drooping or sagging lids early can prevent you from having more surgery later on and can produce great results that last for a long period of time.

Surgery at a Glance

Once you've decided that you are a candidate for eye surgery, consider these preoperative tips:

➤ Don't wear contacts during surgery. Doing so might complicate matters for the surgeon and you won't want to risk losing your contacts. You can begin wearing them again after three weeks with your doctor's permission.

➤ Plan to wear your eyeglasses after surgery for at least a couple of weeks and maybe longer, because pulling on your eyes isn't good for the healing. Your eyes will swell, too, particularly if you've had peeling done. Get used to wearing eyeglasses prior to surgery so you'll be used to them postoperatively.

➤ Decide how much time to take off from work before surgery. You can go back to work in days if the surgery is not a secret and if you can wear dark glasses at work. We recommend that you take at least a few days off, and more if you tend to bruise and swell.

➤ Prepare for surgery in advance. Run all necessary errands ahead of time. You won't want to have to run around after surgery to pick things up.

➤ Plan ahead, and put your makeup away before surgery so you won't be tempted to use it postoperatively. Early use of makeup is not a good idea because it will pull on the scars, particularly when you try to remove it. Postoperative dry spots can grab the makeup, making it difficult to remove.

➤ Buy some Arnica Montana, which is a natural herb that limits bruising, from a health-food store so that you will have it on hand after surgery. You put the tiny wafer under your tongue until it melts into your system. Follow the dosage on the bottle. It is good to use Arnica Montana for a few weeks before and then after the surgery to limit bruising.

➤ Have some zinc and aloe on hand to soothe your skin after your surgery.

➤ Prepare some protein powder and start taking it a week before surgery to add to your building blocks for surgery. Take vitamins, too.

➤ Stay on a low-salt diet before surgery. You don't want to go in to surgery and seem more puffy than you really are.

➤ Know what your medications are and make sure your doctor knows about everything you are taking. It is especially important to avoid any and all anticoagulants, as they can promote bleeding and bruising, and may cause other complications. You won't want to slow down your healing process.

If you follow these tips you'll be better prepared for surgery and have an easier recovery time. It's worth it to plan ahead!

Watch Out!

Now that you've had eye surgery, you're going to want to take extra good care of yourself. Eyelid surgery is different from other surgeries because the swelling, bruising, and any bleeding that happens during your recovery period could temporarily affect your sight. It's going to be very difficult for you to see if your eyes are swollen shut. Here are some simple tips to help you bring the swelling down after surgery:

➤ As noted earlier, it is very important that you avoid wearing makeup until you are healed from surgery. Makeup is more difficult to remove from your eyes right after surgery, and the process of removing it can cause increased swelling.

➤ Most people are tired after surgery. Give yourself plenty of time to rest after your operation.

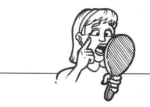

Wrinkle Ahead!

Oral Vite before surgery will contribute to bruising and bleeding, avoid using it postoperatively because it will contribute to wound spread and redness.

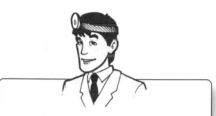

The Doctors Are In

Your recovery time from eyelid surgery will probably be brief if you do not easily bruise because of the quick healing nature of eyelid skin. However, you will need to know where your dark glasses and regular eyeglasses are, and keep your contacts in a safe place so they don't get lost before your surgery.

➤ Elevate your head for the first two weeks after surgery. A 45-degree angle is the least elevation you need. The simplest arrangement is to stay in a chair and prop your feet up on an ottoman.

➤ Remember to get up for food and bathroom and short walks to keep your circulation going. You can wing eye surgery on your own, but if you do business as usual you will have more swelling and take longer to heal.

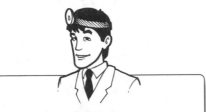

The Doctors Are In

Just because you look good, it doesn't mean you are healed. Follow your doctor's orders and don't risk damaging your surgical results by being too active too soon!

➤ It is not good to fly before the twelfth day after surgery. This can cause complications to your recovery and slow down your healing process.

➤ Don't even think about wearing contacts when you are looking good after a week. You can cause swelling or pull your incisions apart. Try to go three weeks without the contacts.

➤ Keep your hands away from your face and eyes. You'll only irritate your skin and cause more swelling by touching your eyes and the surrounding areas.

➤ Don't get skin ointments into your eyes. This is easily avoided by using them sparingly. Remember, a little bit goes a long way.

If you keep your eyelid surgery a secret, then it's likely that after you have fully recovered from your surgery people will comment on how well-rested and happier you look. That's what we call a successful surgery!

The Least You Need to Know

➤ Eyelid surgery does not make the actual size of your eyes any bigger—it only causes your eyes to appear larger.

➤ Consider having a midface-lift along with your eyelid surgery to improve your appearance even more.

➤ Make sure your doctor doesn't remove too much fat from around your eyes, as this can result in older-looking eyes.

➤ Eyelid surgery does not remedy texture problems of eyelid skin. Texture is a separate issue and should be treated with skin care and peeling, not surgery.

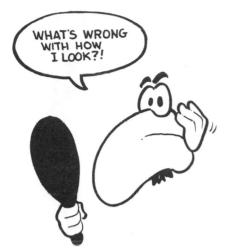

WHAT'S WRONG WITH HOW I LOOK?!

Chapter 8

Follow Your Nose! Nose Jobs

In This Chapter

➤ Understanding the ins and outs of nose surgery

➤ Recognizing the importance of a symmetrical face

➤ How to pick out the nose that's right for you

➤ What you can do to prepare for nose surgery

Let's face it: If your nose doesn't look good, you don't look good. That's why nasal surgery, or what is commonly called a "nose job," has been around since the Renaissance. Fortunately for us, the procedures have improved significantly since those early days, and doctors can now achieve a tremendous level of success when they perform nose jobs. So if you're feeling a bit nosy about what nose jobs are all about, read on!

Knowing Noses

People seek nose jobs to change their noses in a seemingly endless number of ways: to correct a bulbous nose, to make a crooked nose straight, to refine and reduce the size of a large nose, take the point off of a pointy nose, to build up a flat nose. Rhinoplasty really is an art form, and you need to discuss the kind of changes you want made to your nose with your cosmetic surgeon.

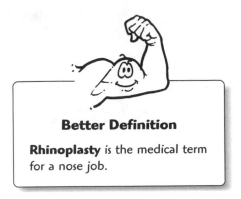

Better Definition

Rhinoplasty is the medical term for a nose job.

You are a candidate for cosmetic nose surgery if ...

➤ Your nose is too wide.

➤ Your nose is too big.

➤ Your nose is too small.

➤ Your nose is too long.

➤ Your nose is crooked.

➤ Your nose is hook-shaped.

➤ Your nose has a bump in it.

➤ Your nose has is pug-shaped.

➤ Your nostrils are flared.

➤ Your nose has a tip that is not the highest point of your nose.

➤ Your nose hangs too low.

➤ The natural shape of your nose has been distorted due to an accident or other trauma.

Today's nasal surgery and its instruments are geared toward creating symmetrical proportions that are functional and natural shadows that appear to be a gift from Mother Nature rather than an imprint from a cosmetic surgeon.

This large nose would be a good candidate for a nose job.

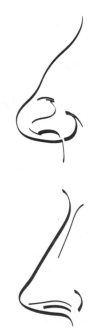

Here's the same nose after surgery. Notice that the size of the nose is the same, but the tip is now delicate and refined.

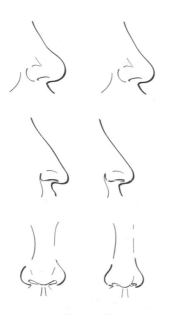

Here are some before and after pictures of various nose jobs.

Putting Your Nose to the Grindstone

Most surgeons and patients agree that the tip of the nose needs to be the highest projecting part of the nose. There also is a universal aesthetic that dictates that the nose should be narrow in most cases. This is often done with chisels or instruments that sand and shape the framework that is underneath your nose.

The Procedures Available

The incisions for nose surgery can either be made on the outside of the nose or on the inside. In closed rhinoplasty, the doctor makes all of the incisions inside of the nose, so the scars will be difficult to detect. In open rhinoplasty, the surgeon makes an incision in the skin between the nostrils. Some doctors prefer open rhinoplasty because it provides better visibility, but most nose jobs can be performed by a skilled physician in a closed procedure, thus reducing the possibility of a visible scar and reducing the amount of postoperative swelling. Nasal surgery gained real popularity starting inthe 1870's when the surgery was done from inside the nose without scars.

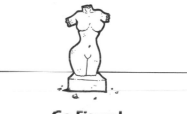

Go Figure!

A need for cosmetic nasal surgery was created in the Renaissance when punishments were doled out on noses. A swordsman would clip the tip of his rival's nose in the course of a duel with his weapon to permanently embarrass the owner of the unfortunate nose. Of course, those who were disfigured in a duel wanted to repair the nose if they could.

The incision for open nose surgery. The scar will be visible when it heals.

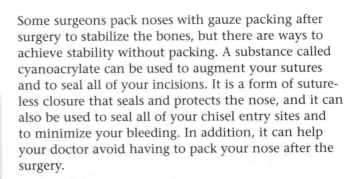

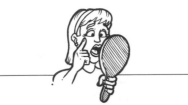

Wrinkle Ahead!

Packing is unpleasant, and its removal is just as unpleasant. Sometimes it is necessary more for respiratory work than for cosmetic work. Talk to your surgeon about options that don't involve packing.

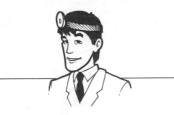

The Doctors Are In

Make sure you discuss the kind of incisions your cosmetic surgeon plans to make. If she or he insists on making an open incision, it might be worth getting a second opinion.

Some surgeons pack noses with gauze packing after surgery to stabilize the bones, but there are ways to achieve stability without packing. A substance called cyanoacrylate can be used to augment your sutures and to seal all of your incisions. It is a form of suture-less closure that seals and protects the nose, and it can also be used to seal all of your chisel entry sites and to minimize your bleeding. In addition, it can help your doctor avoid having to pack your nose after the surgery.

Perfect Imperfections

In the past surgeons would encourage patients to have their noses perfectly straightened, but this is no longer as common. Some doctors even leave a small bump or actually create a small bump in the nose to make the final result look more natural and less surgically produced. More and more people are learning to make some cosmetic improvements, while keeping and becoming happy with their "perfect imperfections"—those distinct characteristics or features that make them unique.

It is still the case, though, that most people place a high premium on narrow nostrils when they consider having cosmetic nasal surgery. However, with more ethnic variety in all cultures all over the world, doctors and patients alike seem to be placing less of an emphasis on removing bumps or imitating a particular ethnic group as an ideal. We think this an excellent idea!

Crooked Noses on Symmetrical Faces

If you have a symmetrical face and a crooked nose, you are the best candidate for a successful nose job. That's because the surgeon can correct the crooked nose and be assured that it will look straight on your face. If your face is already crooked, it becomes very difficult for the surgeon to make the nose look good on your face.

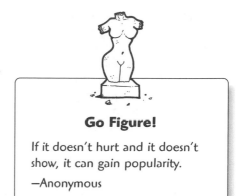

Go Figure!

If it doesn't hurt and it doesn't show, it can gain popularity.

—Anonymous

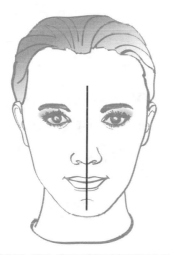

Essentially symmetrical face and nose as seen in full-face view.

Crooked Noses on Crooked Faces

When people have crooked noses and their faces are also asymmetrical, there is no easy solution to their problem. If your face and your nose are asymmetrical, the appearance of both of them cannot be made straight, only improved. Cosmetic surgeons can try to create the illusion of a straight nose with grafting. Grafts can be used to make the nose look more even without moving the bones. This procedure doesn't actually result in a straight nose; rather, it changes the shadows to help create the illusion of symmetry.

When the face is crooked, the center of the eyebrow doesn't line up with the center of the lip, making the nose look crooked. In this case, a nose job might make the nose look even more out of alignment.

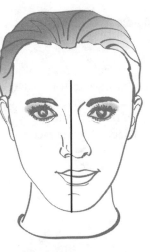

If you corrected the nose on this face, it would end up on one side of the face, making the face appear even more asymmetrical.

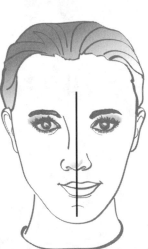

If you are thinking about having cosmetic nasal surgery, consider whether or not your nose is crooked or if your face is noticeably uneven or asymmetrical (keeping in mind that both sides of everyone's face are a little uneven). Then talk to your doctor and get his or her opinion. Discuss your options for cosmetically improving the appearance of your nose.

Cartilage Grafting

If you came into surgery with weak cartilage or other cartilage deficits, it can be replaced during the original surgery with donor material, but this has to be planned for in advance so the doctor can order the material. This approach tends to prevent the need for secondary touch-up surgeries. Touch-up surgeries are frequently required, but they can be limited!

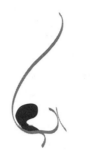

When the tip of the nose is low, such as in this illustration, the nose will need grafts of cartilage or other material in order to raise the tip.

Donor cartilage is a natural substance and heals better than man-made materials that are also used as implants. If you have had silicone implants before, they can also be exchanged for a natural implant during your surgery. This can reduce the risk of your body rejecting the implant or migration of an implant later on.

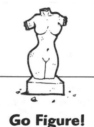

Go Figure!

During the 1920s, some surgeons experimented by placing ivory and other types of bone into noses to create a very sharp, straight, dominant profile. You can see the results of some of these experimental surgeries when you watch the silent-film stars in movies from that era. The reports that were documented from that time did not suggest that patients' bodies rejected the ivory and other natural materials that were used to cosmetically enhance the shape of some noses. This is probably because ivory is a bone and bones are a dead framework that is repopulated with your own cells once it is inserted inside your body.

Be Aware of Limitations

It is important to remember that only so much can be attempted during nasal surgery. A set of priorities has to be established with your surgeon in advance because some goals are more possible to achieve than others. Common complaints from people who have had a nose job and want touch-up surgery include:

➤ The nose is too wide. This can happen when skin does not contract well enough.

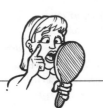

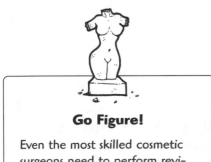

➤ The tip is not crisp enough. This is usually a result from skin that is too thick and weak cartilage. Cortisone injections several months after surgery can help!

➤ There is an unfixable problem that is related to thick skin. Thick skin can be problematic because it may not easily adapt to the framework underneath that the doctor has surgically created during the operation.

If you find yourself in any of these positions, be patient and talk to your surgeon about coming up with a realistic plan of action to achieve the best and most natural look possible.

Unforeseen Complications

Unfortunately, unforeseen complications can occur during this surgery just as with any other cosmetic procedure. When complications arise before, during, or after your nasal surgery, there can be healing issues related to skin contraction (where the skin does not contract around the framework that has been created underneath it), the strength of the cartilage that you were born with, or a graft can be rejected by your body or it can die (if it is your own cartilege or natural substance).

Revision Surgery

As we said in the beginning of this chapter, nose surgery takes a lot of skill, and it is a very challenging surgery. Not everyone is happy with their nose jobs—in fact, less than 50 percent of the people who have nose jobs have revision surgery over a lifetime, to improve upon the original surgery. Make sure you have a candid discussion with your doctor about how he or she handles revision surgeries.

Picking Your Nose (Type, That Is!)

There are some things about your new nose that you want. However, some traits have been predetermined for you already, depending on your skin and features. For instance, if your chin and face is round, a pointed nose will not look natural on you, even if you like it. You will need to pick a nose that has a size and shape that you could have been born with. In other words, the size needs to fit the shape of your face and your other facial characteristics. The nose that your surgeon constructs needs to look like it belongs on your face. Here are some helpful hints to help you pick out your new nose:

➤ **Get some magazines and look at noses.** Identify the noses you like and don't like. Share this with your doctor. See if you can find the ones that look operated on. Remember, not every nose can be done on every person. If the nose you want can't be done on you, it's better to know this before the surgery. If you and your doctor don't agree on what is pretty, it's also better to know this before the surgery.

➤ **Bring photos of what you like to your doctor's office.** It forces you to look at noses in front of your doctor. Ask for your doctor's opinion. If the nose you like is an obvious result of nasal surgery or doesn't fit your face, you need to know this before your surgery. Pay attention to what your doctor thinks is pretty. You need to see at the tip and how it casts a shadow. The natural shadows and the highlights on the tip of your nose are what makes it attractive. You need to take into account the length of the upper lip and how it relates to the nose. Some noses are too narrow or too pointed or have changes in the nostrils that are telltale signs of surgery. You need to see this and avoid it.

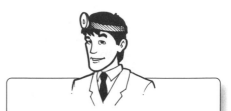

The Doctors Are In

If you think your nose is too prominent, it might really be your chin that is the problem. A weak chin can make a normal size nose appear large. Check out Chapter 9, "Face Your Facial-Implant Options" for information on chin implants.

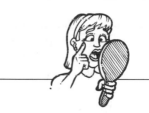

Wrinkle Ahead!

Make sure the person you choose to perform your nose job is a trained cosmetic surgeon who has experience performing nose jobs. Recently in California it was discovered that a dentist was doing nasal surgery!

➤ **Do not get caught up in a computer-imaging program.** They are a nice jumping-off point, but what you see isn't necessarily what you're going to get. Discuss aesthetics with your doctor if you can. Some programs are just that: They do a shrink or rotation but do not take into account what actually can and does happen.

➤ **Ask your doctor where the incisions will be.** If your doctor loves his or her work, he or she will tell you more than you want to know. Be sure that the incisions will be made on the inside of your nose and will be undetectable to others.

➤ **Discuss your doctor's training.** Many people who do good noses don't just do noses, because they are too talented to focus on just one type of surgery. The two boards that train in this field are Ears, Nose & Throat and The American Board of Plastic Surgery.

➤ **Determine if you have a crooked face** that causes your nose to appear crooked from some angles no matter what you do. Remember, a crooked face cannot be fixed; the appearance can only be improved. Feature changes on crooked faces sometimes emphasize the problem rather than fix it.

➤ **Ask yourself: "If I make my nose smaller, will it make my airway smaller?"** There is a limit to how small your nose should and can be. Don't try to set a record. You'll want to look good *and* be able to breathe!

➤ **Know that not everyone heals exactly as they would like to heal.** Following your doctor's orders (before, during, and after your surgery) doesn't necessarily mean your nose will heal in the correct way. Understand that there is always a risk that something can go wrong.

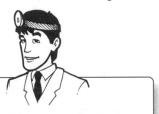

The Doctors Are In

Your doctor should be both inspired and well-trained, and the procedure should be performed in a well-equipped and safe setting. Make sure that a well-trained anesthesiologist will be present throughout the surgery.

When it comes to picking your nose, we suggest you have a cosmetic nasal surgery performed that modifies the structure of the nose you were born with. Even if you want a big change in the size or angle of your nose, there must be something about your nose worth saving. Remodeling your nose can be a lot like remodeling your home. When you remodel your home, you usually leave a wall or some feature, while making larger alterations somewhere else. The same is true with your nose. For your nose to look normal on you, we suggest you keep some of its original foundation and simply add on to its existing structure.

And the Total Is ...

New noses aren't cheap. Expect to pay between $5,000 and $7,000, and perhaps up to $10,000, depending upon the cost of tissue grafts and secondary surgery.

Postnasal Tips

Unlike most other cosmetic surgeries, you cannot easily conceal your nose after you have it operated on. Hair transplants can be covered with a hat, liposuction can be concealed with clothing, and incisions from a face-lift can be covered with makeup.

There is no way to hide your nose! In order to increase your chances of having your nose heal the way it was made and intended to heal, remember the following post-nasal tips after your surgery:

➤ Stay out of the sun.

➤ Avoid bumping your nose with a kiss or a door.

➤ Don't sleep on your side.

➤ Don't wear glasses or even sunglasses from the time the cast is removed until you are three months postoperative. Invest in a good pair of contacts if you haven't done so already and wear them during the three postoperative months.

➤ Steer clear of trauma (and this means no mashing your nose down when you kiss).

➤ Don't go on a mining expedition to clean the inside of your nose with cotton swabs, tissue, your fingers, or anything else! You can pull out the grafts and open incisions that would expose them to the bacteria in your nose. This can cause infection and rejection of your grafts.

➤ Don't stand in the shower or get your cast wet, causing it to fall off.

➤ Stay away from salty food for several weeks after your operation. Salty foods will cause you to swell, and it will slow your healing and might scare you. Don't overeat in the first days because you may be nauseated, and the resulting nausea can create black eyes that you didn't have after surgery.

➤ Don't take your cast off too soon!

Expect to be in a cast for about 12 days. If you take your cast off too soon, there will likely be more postoperative swelling than if you leave it in place for a while. Leaving it on for more than 12 days doesn't help most people. Healing takes a long time (perhaps six to twelve months or more), but you will be presentable after a few weeks, and most people are thrilled to death with how much better they look. There will be days when your nose is more swollen, and the swelling won't completely go away for six to twelve months. (You and other people don't notice the swelling at the time, but a year after surgery, if you review pictures of yourself over the previous 12 months, you'll see the swelling gradually dissipating.) Remember, it takes a year to see the final result, sometimes even 18 months. Barring complications, your nose should heal well and look great over the years. It should age well with you. Sometimes noses need to be touched up over time, but that isn't the case with every nose.

The Least You Need to Know

➤ Make sure you know what kind of nose you want. You may not be able to have it, but from that knowledge you can learn what other possibilities are realistic.

➤ Be prepared for the chance that you will need revision surgery.

➤ Know that noses take quite awhile to heal, so you might not know what the final result will look like for 12 to 18 months.

➤ Avoid the sun after nose surgery at all costs.

➤ Remember Murphy's law applies to the postoperative period; what can go wrong will go wrong—at the gym, at dance class, on a bicycle, and so on. Don't let anyone mash your nose and don't take any unnecessary risks.

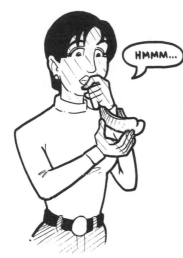

HMMM...

Chapter 9

Face Your Facial-Implant Options

In This Chapter

➤ What facial implant options are available today

➤ How implants in your chin, cheek, and nose can improve your looks

➤ How to determine if an implant will work for you

➤ Making sure you know what you're getting into

Do you have a particular facial feature that you wish was more prominent? Even slight increases in the size of the chin, cheekbones, or nose can make a significant difference in the overall structural appearance of a face. And, as you know by now, good facial structure is the foundation for a beautiful face!

In this chapter, we'll go over the ins and outs of facial implants so that you know what it takes to build a good foundation.

Building a Beauty Foundation

Beauty is in large part fashion, and what is in fashion changes with alarming frequency. Ideal shapes and sizes of features change from season to season and decade to decade. For this reason, we recommend that you carefully consider whether a facial implant is the most appropriate long-term beauty solution for you. As we pointed out in Chapter 1, "Beauty Rules!," there are some internationally recognized standards of

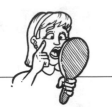

Wrinkle Ahead!

Be careful when considering facial implants to improve asymmetrical features. People with symmetrical features usually get better results from facial-implant surgery. When implants are used to even an asymmetrical appearance, the result often calls more attention to the asymmetry instead of balancing it out.

beauty that have been around for a long time and probably won't change anytime soon. If, after reading this chapter and talking with your cosmetic surgeon, you decide to have a facial implant, we recommend that you get an implant that fits with these standards rather than any particular fashion whim (such as extremely prominent cheekbones) that might be taking the beauty world by storm today. Classic beauty is, well, classic, and it will serve you for a lifetime.

Facial Feature Beauty Standards

Here's a quick recap of some of the international standards for beautiful facial features:

➤ Noticeable cheekbones

➤ A strong chin

➤ A narrow nose with the tip of the nose higher than the nostrils

Facial implants can help to bring your facial features in line with all three of these beauty standards.

Here's a patient who has had cheek implants, a chin implant, and smile lines injected with fat or collagen, giving him a younger, more handsome look. All of these procedures can be done in one sitting.

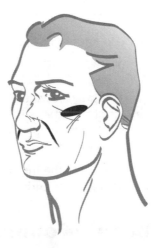

Be a Beauty Conservative!

When choosing a facial implant, we strongly encourage you to take a conservative approach to selecting the size and shape of the implant. Exchanging different-sized implants after they have been surgically inserted into your body is much more difficult than changing your hairstyle.

Chin Up!

Chin-implant surgery has over the last five decades proven to be a successful and well-tolerated operation. You can change the appearance of the entire shape of your face with a chin implant. You can improve your profile by lengthening your chin, or you can enhance your full-face view by squaring off your jaw. Read on to find out about more chin changes.

Chin Changes That Work

You're a good candidate for chin-implant surgery if ...

➤ Your chin is small in profile.

➤ Your chin is too round.

➤ Your chin needs to be squared off.

➤ Your chin is too pointed.

➤ Your chin is oddly shaped from an accident.

➤ You were born with a birth defect or deformity that affects the shape of your chin.

➤ Your jaw is too short.

➤ Your facial features are imbalanced (for example, the shape of your chin isn't in proportion with your nose and cheekbones).

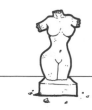

Go Figure!

Before semi-solid silicone and related kinds of implants were developed, injected materials were used to change the shape of patients' features. The first material that we are aware of being injected into patients is parafin. Unfortunately, shortly after being injected, parafin broke down. Even worse, before it broke down, it usually migrated and melted, leaving patients with an unsightly appearance. The parafin would eventually have to be cut out, and this left patients with a permanent deformity!

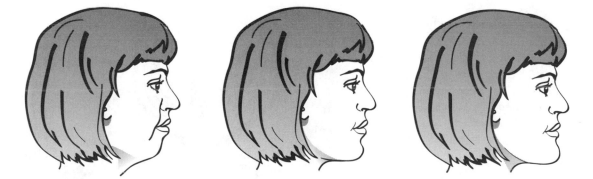

A weak chin, a neutral chin, and a strong chin. See how much of a difference the chin can make to the overall appearance!

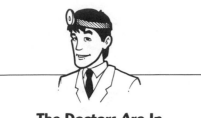

The Doctors Are In

A chin implant can also be inserted during a face-lift. The implant is then usually inserted through the mouth.

The Procedure

Before you actually undergo the chin-implant procedure itself, you will need to consult with your cosmetic surgeon about the size of the chin implant and where it should be placed to achieve the results you are looking for. We strongly encourage you to listen carefully to what size implant your surgeon recommends, and to tell him or her that you would rather err on the size of an undercorrected chin than an overcorrected chin that sticks out too far.

The incision for chin implants is usually made inside the mouth, which means there are no visible scars from the procedure except inside your mouth. The implant is fitted over your chin bone like a dental veneer would fit over a tooth, and it typically holds in place snugly.

Where the incision will be made for chin implant. There will be no visible scars unless someone looks inside your mouth.

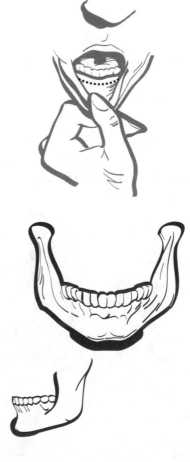

A chin implant fits snugly over the chin bone like a veneer fits on a tooth. It can lengthen the face and balance a face or profile. The chin implant will be permanent and usually does not need to be replaced unless of postoperative complications or injury. The implant can be felt if someone tries hard enough to determine whether or not you've had surgery.

Potential Chin Problems

If your implant is too large for your face, the edges can migrate or be felt or seen from certain angles. In addition, you may run the risk of infection or rejection of the implant, especially if you do not have enough lower teeth or a strong enough chin to hold an implant. We cannot stress enough that if the implant is too big for you it can be a disadvantage and give you an exaggerated look. It is always better to err by having your surgeon undercorrect rather than overcorrect your condition. This is usually a safe, common, and highly satisfactory surgery.

Other than when your surgeon does not recommend an implant (for any reason), the only other condition under which a chin implant should never be used is when you are suffering from an illness that causes deterioration of your chin or jaw. This is typical of some types of cancer. If you suffer from these conditions or any other life-threatening illness, consult with your physician before moving ahead with this surgery or any other cosmetic operation.

Other risks include infection, rejection, and migration of the implant.

The Cost of a Good Chin

A chin-implant procedure, including anesthesia and operating room costs, can run about $3,500 to $4,500.

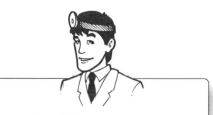

The Doctors Are In

Chin implants come in many sizes, and usually a stock implant will fit most people. However, there are some chin implants that won't fit after a period of time. These are often noted after the first surgery and can be corrected with a custom implant. In rare cases, people with unusual jaw formation will clearly require a custom implant.

Let's Talk About Jaws

Sometimes the jaw is too small for a chin implant or a patient does not want a facial implant. In this case, the jaw can be moved forward. Most jaw problems are more easily corrected if they are treated in early childhood or early adulthood with proper orthodontics. This usually remedies the problem or partially treats the condition of a disproportionate jaw.

As an adult, treatment of a misshaped or disproportionate jaw can be surgically treated with silicone implants or certain bone grafts. Surgery like this is not for the faint of heart at any age, and many people resolve that they would rather learn to accept their appearance instead of enduring the risks and pain of such surgery.

Who Might Be a Candidate for Jaw Surgery

You are a candidate for cosmetic jaw surgery if …

➤ Your upper jaw is shorter than your lower jaw.

Sometimes the upper jaw is too short and can be built up with an implant.

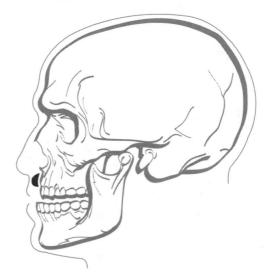

➤ Your surgeon says that your lower jaw is an appropriate size for surgery.

➤ Your lower jaw is too short.

➤ Your lower jaw is too long.

Sometimes the lower jaw is too big and can be trimmed.

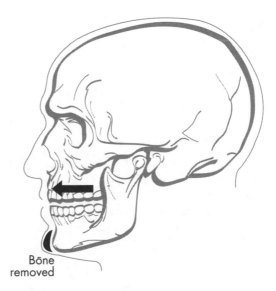

Bōne
removed

➤ Your lower jaw is too angled.

➤ You are willing to consult with orthodontists, maxillofacial surgeons, and plastic surgeons—this is multidisciplinary treatment.

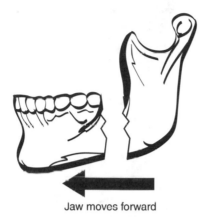

The jaw is cut and moved forward.

Jaw moves forward

You must also be willing to endure a lot of pain and potential risks. Risks include non-unions (bones not healing at all), fibrous union (when bone doesn't heal completely or solidly), and all of the other risks that go along with most surgeries (infection, rejection, and migration, to name just a few).

Jaw surgery is not an operation to enter into without careful consideration. It is a more involved surgery than most cosmetic operations and requires extensive preparation and consultation with other medical professionals. If you decide to have this surgery performed, be sure you remember the risks that are involved and be willing to go the distance! Go to a Plastic surgeon who specializes in maxillofacial surgery or crainiofacial surgery.

Getting Cheek to Cheek with the Facts About Cheek Implants

Cheek-implant surgery is a highly successful operation that usually produces stunning results. Most people who choose to have this procedure performed have cheekbones that are subtle in appearance or almost unnoticeable. Cheek-implant surgery can give some people a younger appearance by restoring the appearance of facial fat that was present in their younger days. Read on to find out all about cheek-implant surgery, then make an appointment with your cosmetic surgeon to get a consultation.

Here is someone with low cheekbones who, with implants, could have a striking face.

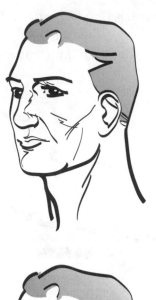

Here is the same person with cheek implants.

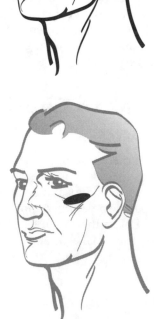

This is where the implants are placed in the face.

Cheek-Implant Candidacy

You are a candidate for cheek-implant surgery if ...

➤ Your cheekbones are too subtle in appearance or unnoticeable.

➤ Loss of facial fat has caused your face to lose its youthful shape.

➤ Your facial features are symmetrical or only slightly asymmetrical.

➤ You have a facial fracture that is in need of restoration.

➤ You have been in an accident that has created a need for reconstructive surgery.

➤ You were born with a facial deformity that could benefit from cheek-implant surgery.

When Surgery Is Not a Good Option

Although cheek-implant surgery can provide stunning results, it isn't effective in some situations. You'll probably want to avoid cheek-implant surgery if ...

➤ You have extremely small or fine facial features, because the implants will look out of place, or they might not adequately attach themselves and end up shifting in your face.

➤ You already have large facial features, because it will result in an exaggerated appearance.

➤ You have asymmetrical cheekbones, because the implant will likely accentuate the asymmetry.

➤ Your cosmetic surgeon suggests that it is unnecessary.

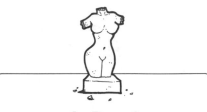

Go Figure!

Cheek implants are often used to re-expand a face that is losing its fatty fill and starting to sag. This is very effective and can have long-lasting effects.

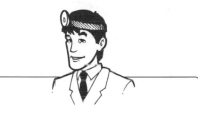

The Doctors Are In

If you have asymmetrical cheekbones, a professional makeup artist might be able to teach you how to apply makeup to address your cosmetic needs. Try this technique first before pursuing surgery.

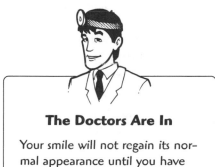

The Doctors Are In

Your smile will not regain its normal appearance until you have had appropriate time to heal, which is three to six weeks.

113

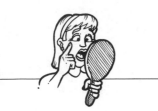

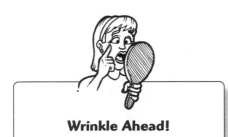

If you have had a facial fracture that did not heal well or left you with an unattractive appearance due to bone loss or repositioning, a single cheek implant may be just what you need. Generally in these circumstances, there is lost fat beneath the eye on the damaged side that makes it appear smaller or sunken. Sometimes correcting the appearance of the cheek with a silicone cheekbone implant can help. However, it can also call attention to this or other problems related to the injury. If you suffer from this condition, ask your surgeon for his or her opinion and discuss whether or not the risk of this surgery would be worth taking.

The Procedure

When cheekbone implants are placed as an independent procedure, they are inserted in the cheek area through small incisions in the mouth. If you are having another procedure such as eyelid or nose surgery, your cheekbone implants also will be inserted through the inside of your mouth. However, if you are having face-lift surgery, they can be placed through your face-lift incisions. They are permanent and will not need to be replaced unless postoperative complications or trauma (a car accident, for example) occurs.

Cheek Charge

Expect to pay around $4,500–$5,000 for a cheek-implant procedure (on both cheeks), including anesthesia and operating-room costs.

Nosing Around

As we discussed in Chapter 8, "Follow Your Nose! Nose Jobs," implants might be required if you want a nose job but don't have enough natural material (including skin, tissue, and cartilage) for your surgeon to work with to create the shape and size of the nose you desire. People who are getting a nose job for the first time and people who were born with minimal amounts of nose cartilage will most likely need an implant to achieve their cosmetic goal. Those who have lost amounts of cartilage, tissue, or skin from repeated nose surgery might also need an implant. We recommend that you nose around to find out if you are a candidate for this surgery!

Natural Implants vs. Semisolid Silicone Implants

Unlike cheek and chin implants, where soft or semisolid silicone gel is the implant material of choice, human donor cartilage are ideal implants for your nose.

Cartilage and bone grafts take longer to heal than synthetic implants. They have the advantage of truly healing into place and becoming part of your body.

The grafts used for this operation might migrate, shrink, or absorb. Your nasal skin will naturally drape and shrink over time, and your final result will not be seen for one year. Sometimes after a year, a minor adjustment of skin or a graft is necessary. This is a safer strategy than trying to have too much surgery performed in one session.

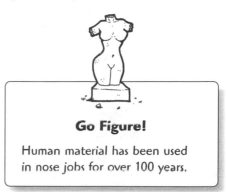

Go Figure!

Human material has been used in nose jobs for over 100 years.

A speedy recovery from this surgery is not a given, and healing will differ in speed and quality from person to person. Also, an agreement between you and your surgeon on the desired goal of your surgery doesn't necessarily mean that you will heal in a desirable way even if everything is done according to plan. Remember, it is a procedure where humans work on humans. Unfortunately, there are no guarantees.

How Much for That Nose?

Noses run $5,000–$10,000, (total) depending upon the donor material and if you have had surgery before. They may be less expensive for first-timers because the surgery is usually less complicated.

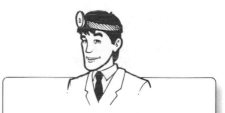

The Doctors Are In

Silicone nasal implants are available and are a viable option for those who want to cosmetically improve their appearance. The risks of using silicone nasal implants are that they can shift or extrude. Natural materials (like your own bone or cartilage) are usually more stable and durable implants over the course of a lifetime.

Preparing for the Face-Off

As you prepare for your facial-implant surgery, there are a few steps that are crucial to practice beforehand.

Pick your anesthesia.

The first step is to discuss with your surgeon what type of anesthesia is going to be used. We highly recommend going with general anesthesia and avoiding local anesthesia, even if it is offered with heavy sedation medications. It is the safest choice of anesthesias and will be more comfortable for you during your operation.

115

Let nature take its course.

Do not be totally fixed on exactly what your result should look like before your surgery. It is important to have an idea of what you want to look like, but remember that outcomes depend on a person's physical makeup and body chemistry. Cosmetic surgery of any kind requires living tissue to heal into a form that nature had not intended it to. Your skin may have a tendency to want to return to its original position and condition. How much memory is built into your tissue and skin is not predictable.

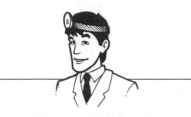

The Doctors Are In

All facial surgeries can result in temporary swelling and numbness that affect muscle function for up to and over one year. These cases are rare but they do occur. Be sure that you are willing to experience this worst case scenario before you have any kind of facial-implant surgery. It's important that you make a fully informed decision.

Anticipate numbness.

With chin and cheekbone implants placed via incisions in the mouth, be prepared to have swelling for some weeks after the surgery that other people won't notice but that will affect your smile. Sometimes you can't smile widely for weeks, even though everything is moving properly. You may even experience some pins-and-needles numbness.

Anticipate seeing your final result in one year for nasal surgery.

Anticipate some minor long-term swelling. Areas affected by nasal surgery and other facial surgeries look swollen to the patient when they don't to others. That is because the patient feels the swelling as well as sees it. There can be minimal swelling in a nose for as long as 12 to 18 months. Usually the swelling is gone in six months, but in some cases it can take up to a year. Your final results will also change and develop as your body changes over the next several years.

Facing Recovery

If you know what to expect after your operation, you will have an easier time during your recovery period. The recovery period for facial surgeries requires a little more precaution than other recovery periods because surgery has been performed around your mouth or nose—two areas that you constantly use each day. Here are some tips to keep in mind during your postoperative period:

➤ Elevate your head as if you were sitting in an easy chair; you'll have to continue this 24 hours a day for the first two or three weeks. Some people find it easier to sleep in a chair with an ottoman to keep their feet up.

➤ A liquid-protein-powder (low in sodium) diet the first two days helps a lot. If you have incisions in your mouth, you need to be on liquids for at least seven days.

➤ Drink fresh fruit juice and protein powder. Canned soup and other canned foods have preservatives and sodium which can make you swell. If you swell, you will worry and be uncomfortable because it stretches the nerves. Eat lightly, but don't starve. You need the calorics to help your body heal.

➤ If you eat too much or eat too quickly, you might get sick. This will bring on bruising and pain, which will slow your recovery. Sip and go slow no matter how thirsty you think you are; in all likelihood, you'll fill up quickly.

Recovery periods are relatively easy and last 12 to 14 days. After you go back to your life, any slight swelling you experience will recede slowly. If you follow these postoperative tips, you should heal very well and be back to your active lifestyle in no time!

The Least You Need to Know

➤ Avoid facial implants if you have an obviously asymmetrical face.

➤ Be conservative when choosing the size of your facial implant.

➤ Make sure you're willing to endure the risks of jaw surgery before undergoing the procedure.

➤ Don't expect to see the final result of any implant surgery for at least one year.

Chapter 10

Pucker Up! Lip Enhancement

In This Chapter

➤ Understanding the ins and outs of lip augmentation and reduction

➤ The pros and cons of liquid injections and sheet implants

➤ Preparing for your procedure or surgery

Whether you're kissing a loved one, sipping an expresso, or talking with friends, you're putting your lips to work. Lips are not only important for going about our everyday lives, they are an aesthetic element of our face as well. Women have long devoted much time and effort to improving the appearance of their lips by applying lipstick and lip liner, and physicians have been using certain cosmetic procedures in order to repair lips after cancer surgery or accidents. However, it is only with relatively recent developments in cosmetic surgery that people have had a chance to change the size and shape of their lips through lip reduction and enlargement for purely cosmetic reasons. In this chapter we will discuss the latest techniques available and explain the pros and cons of lip surgery.

Common Lip Woes

The most common complaint people have about their lips is that they are too thin. People's lips thin naturally with age, but some people just have naturally thin lips. People might also complain that their lips are too full, though because of the latest fashion for, large lips, this isn't as common as it once was.

Lip-Reduction Techniques

People do sometimes have their lips surgically reduced in size, and it is generally a reliable procedure.

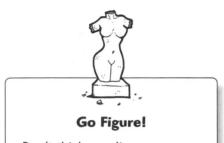

If you are considering having lip-reduction surgery, make sure that your doctor uses a ruler, practices precision care, and doesn't overcorrect your condition by removing too much of your lips. Your doctor can always remove a little bit more of your lip if you are unhappy with your results, but it's very difficult for him or her to increase the size of your lips if too much is removed in the original procedure.

> **Go Figure!**
>
> Don't think your lips are very elastic? Try smiling really wide, then puckering up. Yawn, then frown. That's elasticity!

The Cost of Lip Reduction Surgery

Lip reduction, depending upon the degree, varies between $3,500 and $5,000. This includes anesthesia and operating room expenses.

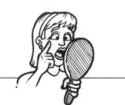

Puckering Up for Lip Augmentation

A mouth stretches and relaxes constantly throughout the day, and cosmetic surgeons have been challenged to find substances that can be added to lips to change their size and shape that will not interrupt the elasticity required for lips to do all they do. Lips also contain many sensory nerves, so it is easy to feel anything that is added to them when you kiss, touch, or eat. Cosmetic surgeons have taken on the challenge posed by lips and have developed nonsurgical and surgical procedures for increasing lip size.

> **Wrinkle Ahead!**
>
> Be sure to "kiss off" any techniques of augmenting your lips if your surgeon wants to eyeball how much of your lip should be augmented, suggests treatment that seems overly aggressive or invasive, or wants to use a technique that is illegal to practice today, such as silicone injections.

It is easier to augment lips that have shrunk with age than it is to create full lips that never existed in the first place. When restoring formerly full lips, the space in your lips is already there naturally. When enlarging lips to a size that you have never had naturally, the enlargement may take more than one session to achieve because of the need to expand a tight and sometimes stubborn space.

Here's an example of how lips empty as we age and do not curve.

Here's an example of youthful lips, which curve.

Lip augmentation material comes in synthetic or natural varieties and is either in liquid or sheet form. We'll discuss each of the kinds in turn below.

Collagen Injections

Collagen is a naturally occurring substance in the skin that is derived from the skin. The use of collagen injections for enlarging lips was developed in the 1970s. By the 1980s, the use of collagen injections was widespread and in part helped create the fashion for full, sensual lips.

In liquid form, collagen is injected into the lips in your doctor's office. The major drawback of liquid collagen injections is that the results are not

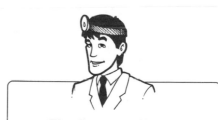

The Doctors Are In

The most common kind of collagen that has been used for several years, is derived from cows and is called bovine collagen. The results of bovine collagen injections are not permanent and must be repeated four to eight times a year.

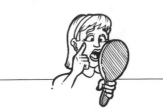

permanent and must be repeated four to eight times a year to maintain full lips. They can also be felt when you kiss!

The Cost of Collagen

Collagen injections typically cost around $500, which includes the cost of the collagen and the doctor's fee for performing the procedure.

Fat Injections

Fat injections are an alternative to collagen injections. The fat is removed from other parts of your body, such as your inner thigh, and is injected into your lips. Fat injections are more permanent than collagen injections, though the fat can be absorbed into the body and thus will likely need to be added to from time to time.

Wrinkle Ahead!

A small percentage of the population is allergic to bovine collagen, so tests must be performed before you receive a full injection of it. Two tests are required with a 30-day waiting period after the first one.

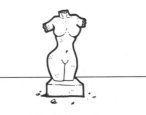

Go Figure!

Injectable collagen replaced the use of silicone injections, which are now illegal and often caused severe and dangerous reactions among patients when they were used in the past.

The Cost of Fat Injections

Fat injections cost less if combined with other procedures, since they are best done under general anesthesia. Done at the same time as other surgery, they cost about $1,500–$2,000. As an independent procedure, it can double because of operating-room costs and anesthesia.

Fat transplants are hard to feel when you kiss, too, but they feel more natural since they actually are a natural part of your body that has been extracted and then reinserted.

Collagen and fat injections must be repeated in order to maintain their results, perhaps every two months to keep up a consistent appearance. As more people have tired of coming back for more treatments, doctors and researchers have started using different substances and have had some luck finding more permanent solutions, which are discussed in the next section.

Alloderm, Fascia, and Gore-Tex

Cosmetic surgeons have started using sheets of natural and synethetic material to create full lips, and while some of them might eventually be absorbed by the skin and need to be replaced, they are proving to be more permanent than collagen or fat injections.

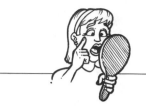

> ➤ Alloderm is collagen that has been derived from human cadavers and formed into thin sheets. It might eventually reabsorb, in which case the surgery would need to be repeated if you want to replenish your lips.

> ➤ Fascia is connective tissue that can be harvested from your own body and reinserted into the lips. It, too, will likely eventually need to be replaced and can be felt when you kiss.

Wrinkle Ahead!

If a fat injection is not done properly, it can result in lumpy or otherwise misshapen lips. Be sure to choose a skilled physician for this procedure.

> ➤ Gore-Tex is a synthetic material. The advantage of Gore-Tex is that it will never be absorbed by the body and thus offers permanent results. The disadvantages are that it is more stiff and might become infected or extrude from the skin, in which case it will need to be surgically removed. It can also be felt when you kiss.

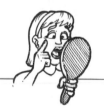

Wrinkle Ahead!

Because Alloderm, fascia, and Gore-Tex as lip implants are all relatively recent developments, the long-term effects are not known. As with any newly developed procedure, you are taking a risk when you choose to undergo it.

When you have synthetic materials put into your face, it's usually not tolerated for more than 10 years, meaning that it may extrude or need to be removed before it extrudes. Certainly there are some exceptions to this, but this is the risk of such surgery. This does not apply to chin and cheek implants.

Having artificial substances used as inserts can lead to unwanted swelling for longer than you might have initially expected, but it usually subsides within a few weeks. Because the insertions are placed in moving areas of your mouth that are naturally

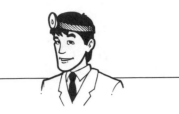

The Doctors Are In

When choosing a physician to enlarge your lips, be sure that he or she takes a conservative approach. The easiest lips to enlarge are those that are to be restored to a size they previously were.

This shows the placement of four different implants in the upper and lower lips. The incisions are made in the corners of the mouth.

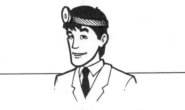

The Doctors Are In

When fat is transplanted, it survives better if done under general anesthesia rather than local anesthesia. It has been said that a local anesthesia effects the metabolism of the fat cell, diminishing its survival rate.

highly unsanitary, the procedure easily lends itself to tearing of incisions, exposure to germs that can cause infection, and rejection of the implants themselves.

The implants are usually placed in four sections of your lips. If one has to be removed or is rejected, you will have to wait for your infection to heal before another one can be inserted. You must weigh the risks involved with sheet insertions and determine whether fuller lips are worth the potential problems. If smaller lips come into fashion at some time, your implants can be removed, but with extreme difficulty and with possible additional complications. Sheet implants are for a person who can evaluate the risks and is willing to take them.

If you are contemplating having your lips cosmetically enhanced, you may want to consider these risks when deciding whether to pucker up and have these techniques performed, or to kiss them off entirely.

The Best Alternative

Collagen injections and fat injections seem to remain the best long-distance runners in the field of lip augmentation because they provide the advantage of no incision and feel more natural when kissing, touching, or eating. They also do not constrain your mouth's range of motion. If there is a problem with your collagen or fat injection that leads to complication, the complication is usually absorption and does not harm you. (Absorption is when your body absorbs the substance). It just takes a little while for your body to

naturally soak up the material and cause it to dissipate. It is an inconvenience leading to disappoint-
ment, but not harm.

Is Lip Surgery Worth It?

Lip surgery requires more than just lip service. You
have to be prepared for your operation. Lip surgery
is going to take time to heal because the swelling
and surgery is right out in front and is not easily
kept clean or concealed. If your doctor used synthetic material to increase your lip size, you already
know that it is not necessarily going to be permanent and will need to be replaced. The decision is
an aesthetic one to compose your features in a way
that is most flattering and enduring for you.

Fashion Trends

Look at the big-lip celebrities and see if their lips
are always big or if they vary. Check out the magazines. Like tattoos, sometimes lip enhancement is
temporary for a shoot. Surgery results are long-
term. If you are following fashion with no greater
commitment than to fashion—which is completely
your prerogative—then do a temporary fix.

Living with Your Decision

Extremes don't last. If you are certain of your real
needs and that you can live with them long-term,
go for a cosmetic procedure if you can live with it
forever. If you want to grow old with it, then move
ahead with your decision. Choose a trained surgeon. As we discussed earlier in this book, this decision is one of the most important keys to getting
a satisfactory result.

Preparing for Lip Surgery

The physical preparation for this surgery is similar to the preparation for other surgeries listed in this book. However, there are some interesting differences. Review the
following preoperative tips:

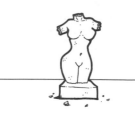

Go Figure!

Unlike other parts of the body
(such as the breasts), foreign material (man-made, not naturally
made by your body) is not necessarily permanent when placed in
the face, because the face tends
to reject foreign materials more
than other parts of the body.

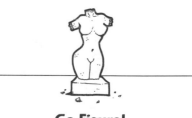

Go Figure!

If you have scars on your lip,
they can be tattooed a natural
pink color. You should always use
a temporary ink that fades in five
years so that if your color and
needs change, you can easily
make the changes. In France, the
law requires that temporary ink
be used for covering scars and
"permanent makeup."

➤ Avoid anticoagulants and salty foods that make you swell.

➤ Be certain you don't have a runny nose brought on by an allergy or cold before surgery.

➤ Consider local or regional block or general anesthesia. (Do you want to be awake?)

Consider these preoperative tips and discuss your options with your doctor. Preparing for lip surgery is just as important as your postoperative recovery period and it is much easier to plan. However, it does require more than just lip service!

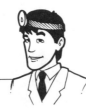

The Doctors Are In

Remember that lip surgery can be repaired but is difficult to undo. You need to know your own mind. If you have very thin lips, the decision might be more easily made than if you have normal lips and just want a little bit more size. Remember, the only one sure thing is that change will occur. In the Renaissance, women shaved their eyebrows and that was the hot look. In the 1920s tweezing to a pencil line was done. The 1960s had some very stylized eye- makeup patterns that some people permanently tattooed in place. All these styles lasted for a while and then were replaced with something quite different. Fashion always changes, and this applies to the large lip size that is currently in fashion. If you think about it, you might decide that it is better to go for conservative, stable good looks that will withstand the test of time, instead of a altering your appearance in such a way that would be difficult to undo when styles change.

Preventing the Kiss of Death

The goal of lip surgery is to create lips "to die for," not lips that could be considered the "kiss of death." You'll want them to heal in such a way that they look smooth and natural to the sight and touch. In order to prevent the kiss of death and achieve great-looking lips that will last long-term, follow our postoperative tips listed below:

➤ Don't eat solid food for a week or two. Maintain a liquid diet.

➤ Take your antibiotics starting the day before surgery and for nine days after.

➤ Ice your lips to reduce pain and swelling.

➤ Avoid hot (heated, not spicy) foods and beverages and hot baths because this can hurt your fat transplant and delay healing in the first days after surgery.

➤ Avoid anticoagulants such as antihistamines and other feel-good over-the-counter medications.

➤ Avoid salt in prepared foods, soups particularly, or you will swell and delay your healing.

➤ Don't kiss your friend or your dog. You won't want to catch anything or get an infection.

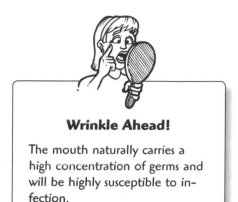

Wrinkle Ahead!

The mouth naturally carries a high concentration of germs and will be highly susceptible to infection.

Lip surgery is considered a fashionable surgery that may quickly go out of style and be less desirable to the population at large, except to those who have under-endowed lips and to those who have lips that have shrunk due to aging. The refilling of aged and aging lips have been a popular treatment and will most likely remain a popular treatment. If you are considering lip-restoration treatment, remember that most surgeons do not use fat to correct lip lines. They only use it to fill lips and restore their natural fullness. Lip lines are usually treated with peeling, appropriate hormone-replacement therapy, and a recommendation for giving up smoking.

If you are following fashion trends, pursue it with cosmetic alterations that are temporary and easily removed. Permanent changes need to be thought through and be made in proportion to your face. Just as dark-red lip color isn't popular as a permanent enhancement anymore, the biggest lips should not be sought out unless it truly improves and balances the appearance of your entire face.

The Least You Need to Know

➤ Don't make permanent changes you are not certain you will like long-term.

➤ If you get collagen or fat injections, plan to have them repeated once every few months.

➤ Be aware of the risks involved with undergoing any new treatment.

➤ Allow several weeks to heal from any kind of lip augmentation that involves surgery.

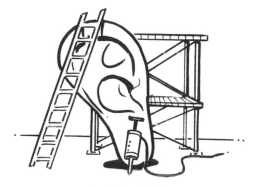

Now Hear This!
Ear Procedures

Ever consider what a normal ear looks like? Probably not. It's usually only by noticing ears that look out of place or misshapen that we begin to identify what an ear *should* look like. In other words, we only notice ears when there is something wrong with them—when they stick out too far from the head, are pointy or otherwise misshapen, or when the earlobes are too small or large.

In this chapter we'll discuss some cosmetic procedures that can be performed to improve the appearance of your ears. The best surgery does not cut the cartilage and ideally leaves a natural looking ear.

Now Hear This!

Even though the vast majority of people who undergo ear surgery do so because of trauma to the ear or severe deformities and birth defects, people also have cosmetic procedures to improve the general appearance of their ears. In this chapter we'll focus on procedures to correct minor naturally occurring ear deformities, not ear deformities caused by trauma to the ear or severe birth defects.

Here's an illustration of an ear. Note that the ear is not flat against the head and that the lobe is not fully attached.

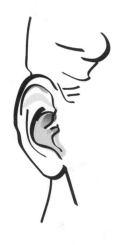

Generally speaking, you can get an aesthetically pleasing result from cosmetic ear surgery today. Cosmetic surgeons can improve the appearance of ears in a number of ways, including ...

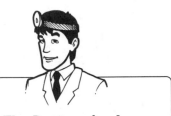

The Doctors Are In

If you can see your whole ear without two mirrors, you are a good candidate for an ear job.

➤ Making large ears into cute curved ones.

➤ Giving pointed ears curved tops.

➤ Creating curves in straight ears.

➤ Attaching ears that stick out too far closer to the head.

➤ Folding the cartilage in what are called "lop ears" (ears that do not have a fold in the cartilage).

➤ Changing the shape or reducing the size of the earlobes.

Here's an ear with a large conch (the top part of the ear that is made of cartilage) and the same ear after surgery to reduce the size of the conch. Note the stepped incision lines in the reduced ear.

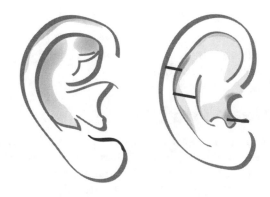

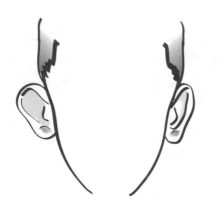

A before and after picture of an ear that underwent surgery for sticking out too far from the head. After it has been set back, the ear still sticks out from the head a little, but this is normal.

Poorly Attached Ears

Set-back procedures are available for otherwise well-formed ears that are not well attached. The surgery involves enlarging the cartilage opening for your ear hole from the inside. You will want to consult with your surgeon about not making the ear hole too big. Getting this just right size is usually an easy procedure. Your doctor will simply trim the extra cartilage to keep the opening to the hearing part of your ear canal the same size.

Lop Ears

Conch or ear-cartilage repairs can be performed for people with "lop ears," or ears where the cartilage did not fold during the course of development. The folds are surgically recreated by your surgeon.

Earlobe Adjustments

If you are unhappy with the size or shape of your earlobes, they can be altered and even reduced in size. Ideally, your lobes should rest at an angle and should not be too attached or rest too close to your head. Lobes need a life of their own so you can flip them to put an earring in.

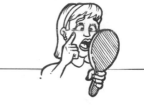

Wrinkle Ahead!

The connection between ear deformity and cardiac and other defects was first noted in the 1960s. Amnioscentesis usually reveals genetic defects, and many fetuses found to have detectable ear deformities today are not carried full term.

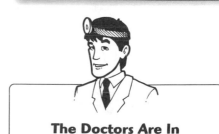

The Doctors Are In

Keep in mind that after surgery you should still be able to see your ears when looking directly into a mirror. Some patients want their ears flat against their head, which is not a natural look.

An ear before and after the lobe has been surgically reduced in size. The ideal lobe should not be fully-attached to the head after the surgery.

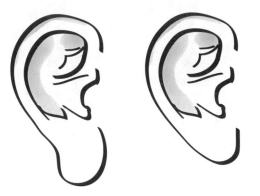

The lobes are trimmed just below the cartilage where they attach to the face.

Your cosmetic ear surgery can be done under local or general anesthesia, and both techniques are routinely performed without complication and are suitable for young children.

The Cost of Ear Surgery

Ear surgery typically costs $5,000, though this can vary depending upon the amount of work required on the ear.

Ear Surgery and Children

Many candidates for corrective ear surgery are children who have decided to have their ears done after repeated teasing from their peers. When children want to have something done about their ears, they usually ask for it. Never push corrective ear surgery on anyone, particularly children. To have a doctor perform elective cosmetic surgery on a child who doesn't want it is an assault of the worst kind.

Children with ear problems generally ask to have something done about them at age five if their ears bother them. This can be done because the ears are fully developed by the age of five. The next age range when the issue comes up again is early adolescence.

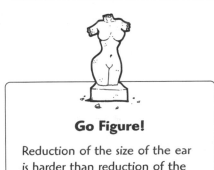

The Doctors Are In

Like snowflakes, no two ears are ever the same. So when you have any type of cosmetic ear surgery performed, expect your two ears to vary a little in appearance.

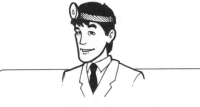

Go Figure!

Reduction of the size of the ear is harder than reduction of the earlobes. It is riskier and can leave scars.

Consider our criteria for candidacy and decide "hear" and now if this procedure is for you or your child. Remember, the person who has the operation has to want it.

Earrings and Ear Problems

People who wear too many earrings or pierce their ears in inappropriate locations might also be candidates for ear surgery. Here are a few tips for how to avoid ear problems caused by earrings:

➤ The upper part of the ear should never be pierced. That area should be decorated with a cuff or a spray in order to prevent damaging or misshaping your ear. Holes in the cupped curved cartilage part of the ear, if infected, can be very problematic and can damage the whole ear; you would need a plastic surgeon who was part magician to get you out of this problem. It would be much better to be safe than sorry!

➤ The lobe, which has a better blood supply than other parts of the ear, is the traditional place to pierce ears. The lobe is also a more resilient area of the ear when it comes to healing in case of infection.

Listen Up

If you've decided to have ear surgery performed, here are some tips for how to take care of yourself before your surgery:

➤ Wash your hair. It's not necessary to cut it for surgery because it can be taped out of the way.

➤ Make sure that you are happy with your hair color before surgery because you won't be able to color it again for three weeks.

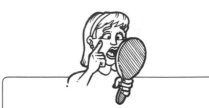

Wrinkle Ahead!

If you are a parent and want your child to have this surgery but your child does not, then you have the problem, not your child. Instead of pushing your child to have the surgery, try working on accepting your child and tolerating the appearance of his or her ears. A little bit of acceptance goes a long way with building a close and loving relationship with your children.

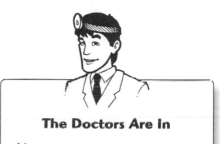

The Doctors Are In

Never suggest an operation to anyone who doesn't want surgery. If they are too young to want it, they are too young to have it. Keep this in mind if you are tempted to talk your children into having cosmetic surgery.

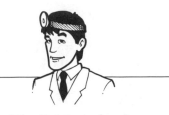

➤ Get lots of rest, eat a high-protein diet, and try to feel relaxed about your procedure.

➤ Arrange to have someone to drive you to and from appointments because the big padded dressing will make it hard for you to hear.

➤ If you wear glasses, find some old or cheap frames because they will get bent out of shape going outside the bandage. You do not want to dig the frame of your glasses into your ears, as it can affect how your upper ears heal.

➤ Be prepared for the fact that your surgery might not be as successful as you'd like and you might need to have it touched up.

Now Hear This!

Once you've made it through your surgery, it's time to gear up for your recovery. If you want to heal as quickly and as smoothly as possible, take our recommendations listed below:

➤ Continue taking your antibiotics, which should have been prescribed to you beginning the day before your surgery. This is very important because it will prevent infection and other complications from arising.

➤ Keep your head elevated and sleep on soft pillows under your back. Have ice ready in waterproof bags in case of pain.

➤ Have your pain-pill prescription available, but as a first line of defense try taking Tylenol or a codeine-type preparation.

➤ Plan on staying home, reading, or watching TV with the volume up. You should be comfortable.

➤ Keep your dressing on for the time period required (usually a week).

➤ Do not roll over on your side—it will hurt!

➤ Use something as a protective sleep band for three months after the surgery; a good choice is ear warmers that you can find at ski shops. A band will protect your ears from the pillow in case you roll over onto your side.

➤ Don't let anyone touch, kiss, or tug on your ear for about three months.

Be sure to follow all of these postoperative suggestions for an idiot-proof recovery!

The Least You Need to Know

➤ Consult with your doctor about changing the shape, size, or position of your ear.

➤ Don't push ear surgery on your children if they don't want it.

➤ Be prepared to undergo a second procedure in order to get the desired effect.

➤ Keep your head elevated after surgery in order to speed up the recovery process.

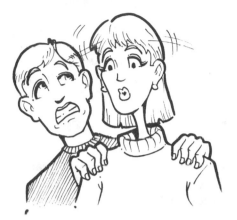

Chapter 12

Let's Neck! Neck Liposuction

> ### In This Chapter
>
> ➤ Recognizing the role the neck plays in making you look old or young
>
> ➤ How neck fat contributes to wrinkling and drooping
>
> ➤ Discovering the miracle of neck liposuction
>
> ➤ Finding out if you're a good candidate for neck liposuction
>
> ➤ The cost of a new neck

Whether you're a man or a woman, your neck has a profound effect on how young or old you look. Unfortunately, you can't look young if your neck is heavy and doesn't have clean, smooth lines, even if you have a young-looking face. And if you are young and have a naturally fat neck, you will have a tendency to look older than your actual age and out of shape no matter what condition the rest of your body is in. It's almost impossible to look young or lie about your age when your neck has a life—and look—of its own.

In Chapter 5, "Turning Heads and Breaking Hearts: Face-Lifts," we discussed the traditional neck-lift surgery, which is usually done at the same time as face-lift surgery. In this chapter we'll show you what you can do to improve the appearance of your neck with liposuction procedures, or what we call neck sculpting.

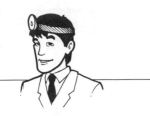

Many necks that are fat, droopy, and wrinkled are just pulled downward by the excess weight of fat. If the skin has enough elasticity in it, such necks can respond well to liposuction procedures, and once the fat is removed the skin will contract naturally. This can have a tremendous impact on someone's overall appearance, making them appear more youthful and fit.

The Miracle of Liposuction

Liposuction is a minimally invasive surgery. A very few small incisions need to be made, and they can be placed in strategic areas away from the neck so that the scars are almost undetectable when you heal.

The Doctors Are In

Liposuction works best for people who diet and exercise but are unable to get rid of diet-resistant fat. Facial and neck fat is hard to gain back after liposuction. It is not impossible, but it is uncommon.

Before your surgeon actually sucks out your excess fat, he or she will inject a fluid into the area to be treated that will control bleeding, making it easier to suck out. The doctor will then insert a narrow rod that is attached to a suction machine or syringe and will suck out the fat. After your surgery, you will likely be asked to wear a tight bandage around your neck and head to aid in healing and skin contracture.

The two common incision sites for a neck liposuction procedure. The scars are usually well-hidden once healed and will be small.

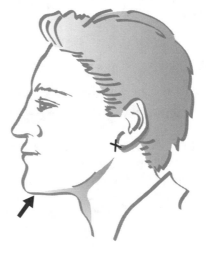

Neck Liposuction Candidates

Liposuction of the neck is most effective on people who have good skin tone but excess fat. The following are a description of neck problems that are candidates for neck liposuction:

➤ Born fat: People who were born with fat pads in their neck that didn't recede as they should have over the course of physical development are perfect candidates for liposuction.

➤ Midlife fat: Liposuction can also benefit people who developed these fat pads in middle life (in their 40s) along with fat pads on other parts of the body.

➤ Short jaws and large necks: Although short jaws and large necks are not totally improved by this surgery, their appearance can often be improved upon. If your jaw is short, your skin will tend to droop sooner than someone who has a longer jaw because it has less of a structure to support it, and you will look older more quickly than someone who has a larger jaw. The results of surgery won't be as dramatic as if you had a large jaw, so we recommend that you discuss other options with your cosmetic surgeon.

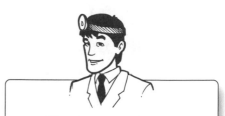

The Doctors Are In

If your jaw is weak (i.e., small or short), the fat may be more of an illusion and due to muscle sag instead of the presence of real fat. Liposuction is not always the best remedy for this problem. Jaw advancement can help. It is for the very young—ages 18 to 25, because younger people tend to heal well enough for this procedure.

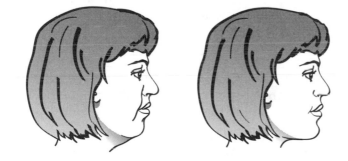

Before and after pictures of someone who had neck liposuction. Notice the dramatic improvement.

The Importance of Youthful Skin

It is important to note that as you get older, skin contraction becomes less likely, and by age 40 or so, some people's skin will not contract well enough with liposuction alone. If this is the case, they will probably need a traditional neck lift (see Chapter 5) in addition to liposuction. We do recommend that if you are heavy or have extra fat pads around your neck, you should have this surgery performed sooner rather than later. The surgery seems to last a long time and may delay future sagging caused by the fat pulling your skin of your neck downward.

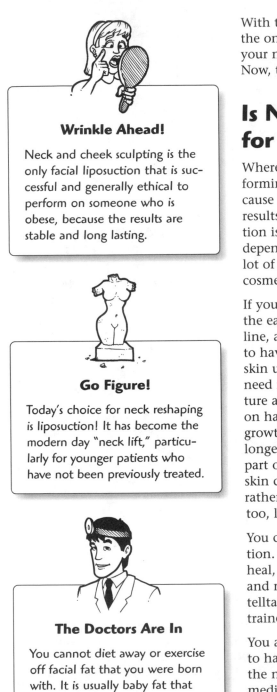

Wrinkle Ahead!

Neck and cheek sculpting is the only facial liposuction that is successful and generally ethical to perform on someone who is obese, because the results are stable and long lasting.

Go Figure!

Today's choice for neck reshaping is liposuction! It has become the modern day "neck lift," particularly for younger patients who have not been previously treated.

The Doctors Are In

You cannot diet away or exercise off facial fat that you were born with. It is usually baby fat that failed to involute and can only be surgically removed.

With the proper use of today's liposuction techniques, the only person who might know that you've had your neck resculpted—besides you—is your surgeon. Now, that's what we call a great surgical result!

Is Neck Liposuction Right for You?

Whereas many surgeons only feel comfortable performing neck lifts in conjunction with face-lifts because the surgery is easier to perform this way and the results are more aesthetically pleasing, neck liposuction is performed in large volumes as a procedure independent of face-lifts. You don't even need to have a lot of fat to have your neck and chin fat corrected by a cosmetic surgeon.

If you are fully grown—18 in females, 19 in males (at the earliest)—you can suction out your neck, your jawline, and perhaps some cheek fat. Youth who choose to have surgery tend to respond well because their skin usually contracts well and it may even delay the need for a face-lift later in life. Some kids are more mature and can shave a few months off these ages based on hand X-rays that show that they are basically full growth. This type of liposuction works better (and longer) when performed on a young patient, because part of aging is the weight of the fat pad that pulls the skin down. Sometimes the fat is under the muscle rather than between the skin and muscle, and this, too, lends itself to suction techniques quite easily.

You don't need a lot of neck fat to have neck liposuction. The less fat that is suctioned, the less there is to heal, but there are exceptions to this rule. Most major and minor liposuction surgeries heal well and without telltale signs of surgery when performed by well-trained hands.

You also do not need to have a lot of neck fat in order to have your neck suctioned because liposuction of the neck can be used as a preventative method. Most medical experts believe that the fat pulls the skin down, and takes the muscles down with it. If you treat this condition early with proper liposuction, you may be able to delay or spare yourself from having a face-lift later on. You don't want to have too much fat removed from your face or you will look harsh later on.

How Much for a New and Improved Neck?

Neck liposuction isn't cheap, but many people think it's worth it. Expect to pay around $4,200 for a full neck and cheek liposuction.

Preparing for Neck Surgery

Having any surgery requires some basic preparation. Even though you will feel well most of the time, you will probably want to rest quietly at home because you will be wearing a tight bandage on your head after your surgery, and you will experience some swelling. For these reasons, we suggest that you prepare ahead of time for your surgery. We recommend that you plan for your comfort and to have plenty of activities available to keep yourself occupied—reading, watching TV, listening to music, or surfing the Internet.

Most people fall asleep easily and experience sudden fatigue after surgery, so don't plan activities that require deep concentration or extreme amounts of physical activity. Here are some common preoperative tips to help you become prepared for your neck-resculpting operation:

➤ Set up pillows so you can elevate your head. Ideally, you need to keep your head up to control swelling for as long as 10 to 14 days.

➤ Prepare cold compresses and keep them available just in case a headache occurs. A cold compress is good treatment for a headache and can help to reduce the amount of pain medication that you need.

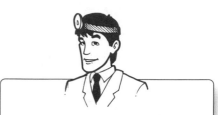

The Doctors Are In

People who enjoy outdoor activities and hobbies usually experience moderate to severe sun damage to their necks if they have not used sunscreen. Sun damage can cause a neck to wrinkle prematurely and can cause you to look much older than your actual age. Liposuction can't help sun-damaged skin but there is advanced skin care available today that may help and peeling that can be performed by a skilled practitioner.

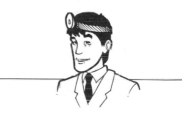

The Doctors Are In

Some people can diet away neck fat and keep it off if they have a normal to fast metabolism, practice self-restraint, and maintain an active lifestyle. Other people who are unable to diet away neck fat and naturally have heavy necks will need to have surgery performed.

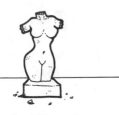

Go Figure!

Necks were first suctioned in the 1980s, and these patients are still doing well.

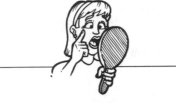

Wrinkle Ahead!

If you think your neck needs to be suctioned but your surgeon is unable to see what you see, take our friendly advice: Don't expect a doctor to operate on what he or she cannot see, feel, or photograph. If your doctor cannot see it, feel it, or photograph it, it would really be impossible for him or her to operate on it, and you won't want to pay real money to have an imaginary and unnecessary surgery performed. Your money just might be better spent on counseling to better understand and cope with your different view of your body.

➤ Arrange to have someone stay with you to answer your phone and doorbell, or rig these devices so that they light up when they ring. It is hard to hear with bandages on your head.

➤ Plan ahead! You'll need someone to drive you to and from the doctor's office. Later, you'll also need someone to drive you to your doctor's office for a postoperative checkup because you won't be able to turn your head.

A speedy and problem-free recovery will depend on proper preparation. If you plan ahead, you can also plan to have a successful recovery!

Necking No-No's

After your neck surgery, there are a few things to remember *not* to do—we call these "necking no-no's" because they will have an adverse effect on your surgery, cause possible complications, and slow down your recovery period. The most important necking no-no to remember is to avoid eating solid food for the first few days after your surgery. We recommend that you maintain a liquid diet because the less you chew, the less you will swell after your surgery. Other factors that cause swelling are salt and preservatives. Soups and foods that are bottled or canned tend to contain these ingredients and should be avoided as much as possible in order to maintain an uncomplicated recovery period.

You will be wearing a compression dressing that will help your skin to contract and form to the underlying structures and help minimize bruising for the first few days of your recovery period. Consuming foods and other ingredients that induce swelling can prevent skin contraction and swelling reduction. Here are some other important postoperative tips that we think would help your recovery period to go as quickly and as smoothly as possible:

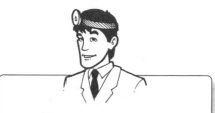

➤ Moderate walking is OK, but don't engage in a lot of physical activity.

➤ Elevate and ice your head so you don't have swelling and pain.

➤ Don't forget your medication! Take few pain pills, or try starting with Tylenol first—it should be enough to reduce your pain without the need for prescription drugs.

➤ Don't take off the bandages to peek at your results. This can cause complications to arise and slow down your healing process.

➤ Don't try to drive with big bandages in place. It is a danger to yourself and others.

The Doctors Are In

Buy a small handheld calendar to keep a schedule of when you take your antibiotics. This isn't a good time to forget them.

➤ Don't wet your bandages. Shower from your neck down. Shampooing your hair can wait until later.

➤ Don't be unattended. It is very easy to fall on stairs or in a bathroom. Have someone with you at all times!

➤ Recovery is usually not uncomfortable, but facial dressings can be cumbersome.

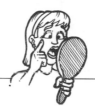

Wrinkle Ahead!

There are untrained doctors reading books and doing direct excisions on patients, which most cosmetic surgeons stopped performing years ago. Be sure to check out your surgeon's training and credentials. You'll want a surgeon who is properly trained (certified through the American Board of Plastic Surgery), has vast experience in performing neck surgery, and uses the most up-to-date techniques. Avoid experimental procedures unless you are well informed of the dangers and are willing to take the risks.

When doctors and patients think of neck liposuction and the recovery period, they think of it fondly. Most patients and their doctors are very happy about the results of this procedure. The healing phase varies but tends to be fast. This type of surgery is very long-lasting and can delay—if not prevent—a need for a face-lift. This surgery does not create eternal youth, but it is can become an important building block for maintaining a youthful appearance.

143

The Least You Need to Know

➤ Make sure your skin is young enough that it will contract after neck liposuction.

➤ Consider neck liposuction in combination with other procedures operations (such as a face-lift) to maximize your results and minimize your recovery period.

➤ Avoid salty foods or foods with preservatives after surgery in order to reduce swelling.

➤ Keep the bandages on for one full week, and no peeking!

Chapter 13

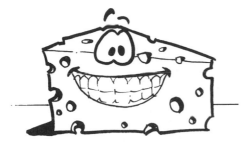

Say Cheese! Cosmetic Dentistry

In This Chapter

➤ What you can do to whiten and brighten your teeth or straighten out your smile

➤ How dentists are focusing on conserving teeth and enhancing their beauty

➤ Ways to improve your smile and how much it costs

➤ Taking care of yourself after your procedure

It seems like everyone from your neighbor down the street to your favorite super-model is in search of the whitest and brightest choppers. And there's good news in the field of cosmetic dentistry for all of us who want to have flashy pearly whites: Medicine and technology in this field can now give almost anyone a better and brighter-looking smile. Most of us are only a few procedures away from having a beautiful smile.

In the past, techniques that improved the appearance of your smile usually involved the removal of some teeth or other painful procedures. Now smiles can be improved in numerous other ways.

Ways to Improve Your Smile

There are so many ways to improve your smile! Some procedures are better than others for improving size and shape, while others are better for improving color or overall appearance. Knowing which procedures are most commonly used to improve

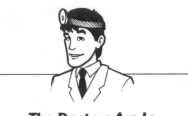

The Doctors Are In

Knowledge *is* power. Learn as much as you can about the various dental procedures before visiting your cosmetic surgeon.

particular imperfections will help you to make an informed decision about which procedure would best fit your cosmetic need:

➤ You can restore the size and shape of your teeth with bonding.

➤ You can reduce the appearance of your gums and have a bigger smile with gum reshaping.

➤ You can even out your teeth with teeth reshaping.

➤ You can brighten your smile with teeth bleach.

➤ Or, you can completely change the appearance of your entire smile with veneers.

Bonding

Bonding is the cosmetic procedure of applying white-colored plastic to a patient's teeth. This is usually done to fill in chipped teeth, fill in small gaps between teeth, or to whiten teeth by masking difficult stains. Bonding is a quick and simple procedure that can be done in your dentist's office. Since it causes very little if any discomfort, anesthesia is usually not needed.

Estimated cost: $135–$360 per tooth.

Gum Reshaping

Gum reshaping is a cosmetic procedure that improves "gummy smiles"—those smiles in which the gums are overly prevalent. During gum reshaping, the patient's gums are surgically separated from the upper and lower front of the teeth (usually just the front eight to ten teeth on the top and bottom—if both sets need it). The upper and lower front of all teeth are then filed in such a way that causes the gums to rest higher up and lower down on the teeth than before. Once the gums are reattached, the patient is left with a smile that reveals more teeth and less gum. The teeth look longer and the gums look shorter.

Anesthesia is required for this operation and stitches are used to suture the gums. Recovery takes seven to ten days. General pain, swelling, and bleeding can be expected.

This operation should only be performed by an oral surgeon.

Estimated cost: $950–$1,100 per tooth.

Teeth Reshaping

Teeth reshaping is a quick and easy procedure that can be performed in a matter of minutes. The procedure involves the use of an electric sander to gently and quickly sculpt the shape of your teeth. It can be used to smooth small chips in teeth, even out inconsistent teeth length, slightly decrease the amount of enamel on the front of protruding teeth, and give patients a more gender-specific smile.

This procedure is relatively pain-free and does not require anesthesia.

Estimated cost: About $125 per tooth.

Teeth Bleaching

Bleaching the teeth to lighten the look of stained or discolored teeth is a popular and relatively inexpensive way to improve your smile.

An initial consultation is required to take an imprint of your teeth, from which a mold of your mouth will be made to create plastic trays that will fit over the top and bottom rows of your teeth. These trays will be filled with a teeth-bleaching solution. Solutions usually come in different strengths, and your dentist will most likely begin with the mildest solution to test your teeth for sensitivity to the bleach. The bleach will only lighten the enamel of your teeth; it will not have an effect on your dental work (such as bonding or veneers).

You will likely need a series of teeth-bleaching treatments to achieve the degree of whiteness you desire. Six months to a year after that, occasional follow-up visits may be needed. Teeth bleaching can be done in the office or at home. At-home teeth bleaching should be performed under the direction of your cosmetic dentist. Follow-up treatments are usually much less expensive than the initial visit.

Estimated cost: $200–$300 for all teeth.

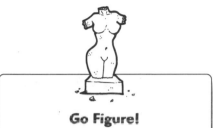

Go Figure!

Did you know that men's and women's teeth have different characteristics? Characteristics of a feminine smile are teeth that are smaller and have a more rounded shape. Characteristics of a masculine smile are larger, square-shaped teeth. Teeth reshaping can help men and women achieve more gender-specific looks.

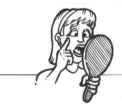

Wrinkle Ahead!

Avoid teeth staining foods such as coffee, teas (hot and iced), berries, tomotoes, red wines, and dark colas to keep your teeth looking their whitest and brightest. Also, avoid smoking of any kind.

147

Veneers

Veneers are porcelain facades that are fastened to the front of the teeth with adhesive. Unlike caps, they do not require that the size of your tooth be drastically reduced and they do not surround the entire tooth. These porcelain facades come in a variety of tooth-colored shades, shapes, and sizes. Anesthesia is commonly used during this procedure and there is no recovery time. Veneers are very effective in giving anyone and everyone the appearance of a brighter and bigger-looking smile! It is a very common procedure with a very high success rate.

Estimated cost: $800 per tooth.

Preparing for Your Dental Procedure

The old adage, "If you fail to plan, you plan to fail," applies here. You'll need to do your homework before seeing your cosmetic dentist, and that means knowing what to expect before you even walk through the door of his or her office.

In the next section we'll tell you exactly what will be required of you before you decide to have any of the aforementioned procedures performed.

If any of the dentists you visit do not recommend any of the following suggestions, be sure to ask them why or why not. In the interest of your safety and physical health, most cosmetic dentists will insist on the following.

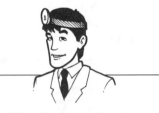

The Doctors Are In

All cosmetic improvements made to your teeth require professional inspection and cleaning. This will reduce the risk of infection, cavities, or other complications during or after your procedure. Be sure to have your teeth professionally cleaned by your dentist before any cosmetic improvements are made.

Initial Consult

Most cosmetic procedures require an initial consult with your dentist so that you can discuss your cosmetic goals; the dentist then will recommend a procedure and explain how it will be performed. It is important to remember that these are your teeth and any cosmetic improvement made to them is 100 percent your choice. Be sure that your dentist fully understands your needs and that you feel completely comfortable with the cosmetic procedure that you ultimately choose.

A Full Periodontal Evaluation

During your initial consult, you should receive a full periodontal evaluation. Your cosmetic dentist will evaluate your teeth for cleanliness, cavities, chips or cracks, tooth mobility (to see if any of them move), and quality of gum tissue (to see if you have gum disease). He or she will evaluate the supporting structure of your teeth (the base of your teeth) for stability. Your periodontal exam may also include x-rays. Keep this in mind, and be prepared for a full periodontal evaluation before your cosmetic procedure.

Knowing what will be expected of you before you choose a cosmetic procedure will help you to feel more relaxed and plan ahead. If your doctor requests that you do any of these things—the periodontal exam, x-rays, a teeth cleaning—know that he or she is not trying to run up an unnecessarily large bill. Your doctor is only doing his or her job and taking every precaution that is required to give you top quality care.

What Happens Next?

So, what happens next? Now that you've learned about your options, decided which alternative is best for you, and you've actually had the procedure done, what can you expect? The answers are surprisingly simple.

You can return to work the same day.

All cosmetic procedures (with the exception of gum reshaping) performed in your dentist's office have little to no recovery time. Most dental improvements can be made quickly and with little to no discomfort. Usually anesthesia is not required. This means that you can return to work or your regular daily activities immediately after your dental appointment.

Your teeth may be sensitive.

Many of the dental procedures that improve the appearance of your smile can cause some mild and immediate forms of tooth sensitivity. Know that this is a normal reaction that will be only temporary. The feeling should not last longer than a few days and usually dissipates much sooner than that. If your teeth continue to feel extremely sensitive even after a few days, contact your dentist.

Avoid extremely hot or cold foods and beverages— ouch!

Avoid extremely hot or cold foods and beverages if you are experiencing tooth sensitivity after your dental procedure. When tooth sensitivity occurs, the nerves in your teeth are very receptive to extreme temperatures. Hot or cold items can cause major discomfort to your teeth and to other areas of your mouth.

No crunching!

Avoid eating hard, crunchy foods if your teeth still feel sensitive after you've left your dentist's office. Whole apples, corn on the cob, granola, and other similar foods will be difficult to eat and can cause minor to major discomfort for the first few days after your procedure. If you've had veneers put on your teeth, you will want to permanently avoid these foods, as they may cause your veneers to pop off.

Just say "no" to staining agents.

To keep your teeth and your dental work looking their whitest and brightest, avoid agents that will stain your teeth. Teeth-staining agents include coffee, tea, red wine, dark sodas, juices, berries, and, of course, smoking. All of these agents will cause your teeth to darken and dull prematurely. They also permanently stain most dental work.

Don't forget to brush regularly.

Maintain the cleanliness and brightness of your smile by brushing your teeth regularly after every meal. If you work full-time and are unable to go home for lunch, bring your toothbrush and toothpaste to work and be sure to keep your smile looking white and fresh all day long. It may sound inconvenient, but practicing proper dental hygiene at work will probably be more convenient and less expensive than having to have a cavity filled because you did not brush your teeth regularly.

Stimulate those gums!

Stimulating your gums can help to promote healthy blood flow throughout the gums and help to prevent gum disease. You can stimulate your gums by massaging them with a toothpick or an over-the-counter gum stimulator, which is available at most drugstores and pharmacies.

Always floss ... always, always, always.

Never underestimate the power of flossing! Flossing will help to keep your teeth radiant and your smile looking its absolute best. Besides, it helps to prevent cavities. Always floss. Always!

So what are you waiting for? You're only a consultation away from knowing what you can do to improve your smile!

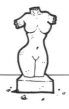

Go Figure!

Cosmetic dentists all are focusing on ways to improve people's smiles without needlessly extracting teeth or reducing tooth size. Dr. Michael Delmont of Cedars Sinai Hospital in Beverly Hills, CA, notes, "Greater tooth conservation will be the main focus of most forms of dentistry, including cosmetic dentistry. Also, more and more dentists are using a 'team approach' when it comes to improving patients' smiles. They are consulting with oral surgeons, orthodontists, and other dental experts to come up with alternative ways of improving people's smiles while still maintaining the quality of their teeth."

The Least You Need to Know

➤ Ask your dentist about alternative methods of improving your smile or quality of your teeth besides tooth extraction or drastic reduction of tooth size.

➤ Allow tooth extractions and drastic reductions of tooth size only as a last resort.

➤ Be sure that your cosmetic dentist fully understands your needs.

➤ Get a full periodontal evaluation before any cosmetic dental procedure is performed.

Part 3

Better Breasts and Chests

Breast augmentation, breast reduction, and pectoral implants are all upper-body proce-dures that should be entered into only after careful consideration. Each of these surger-ies can improve your appearance by producing almost irreversible results. Implants create semipermanent to permanent results, you will want to consider carefully whether or not you want to proceed with these figure-altering and physique-changing operations. If you change your mind, the outcome will be difficult to undo.

Most people who elect to have these operations performed are happy with their results. They don't even mind having the implants removed or replaced when they wear out or need to be changed later in life. They believe that it is an improvement worth making and plan to have future surgeries performed in order to maintain their results when-ever it is necessary. They know that most implant surgeries will usually require a maintenance surgery sometime in the future and consider the additional procedure an investment worth making!

Chapter 14

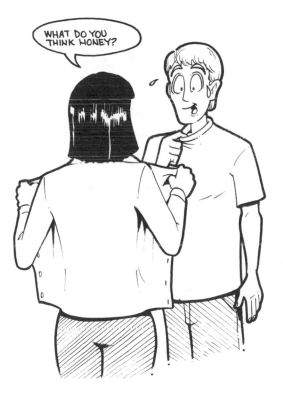

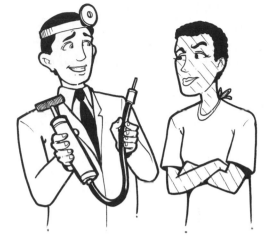

Busting Up!
Breast
Augmentation

In This Chapter

➤ How to determine if breast implants are right for you

➤ Understanding implants

➤ The ins and outs of incisions

➤ What to ask your doctor in an initial consult

Are you on a quest for bigger breasts? You're not alone! While women strive to rid fat from their fannies, hips, and thighs, thousands, if not millions, of women wish they could add a few ounces of flesh to their breasts. And although some breast-enlargement techniques have come under fire in recent decades, there are many safe and effective procedures for increasing the size of your bust.

The Biggest Isn't Always the Best—But Sometimes It Is!

Not every woman who is curious about breast enlargement wants to end up with large and conical breasts like Jane Russell's ... although some do. Women with breasts that barely fill an A cup might be hoping to fill out a C cup after their surgery. Other women who already have moderate-sized breasts might want firmer and only slightly fuller breasts. And, of course, there are women who desire very large breasts.

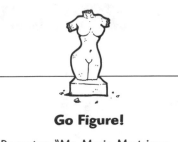

Go Figure!

Reporter: "Mr. Mario Mastrione, how is it that Miss [Sophia] Loren is paid a million dollars for a movie, and you are paid only one hundred thousand dollars to costar in the same movie?"

Mr. Mastrione: "Breasts are breasts."

—Interview with Mario Mastrione, Italian movie star

The Lay of the Land

Not everyone is a good candidate for all kinds of breast-enhancement procedures. One way doctors determine what procedure might be most appropriate for a patient is to look at where her nipples fall in relation to the crease under the breasts. You can do this at home: Without a shirt or bra on, stand up straight and look at your profile in a mirror. See the fold under your breasts? That's called the inframammary crease, and where your nipple falls in relation to the crease is a good indicator of what procedures will be effective for you. Once you've taken note of whether your nipple is above the crease, at the level of the crease, or below the crease, read on to see what procedure might be best for you:

➤ If your nipple is above the crease, you are a good candidate for breast augmentation and will likely have excellent results from breast-implant surgery.

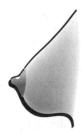

The nipple on this breast is well above the crease, making the breast ideal for implant surgery.

➤ If your nipple falls level with the crease line, you are not an ideal candidate for breast augmentation, but a large implant can increase the size of your breast and lift them up so they don't droop so much. However, drooping can reoccur at any time and the breasts will likely need to be re-done over time.

This nipple is level with the crease. A large implant will increase the size of the breast and give it a little lift.

➤ If your nipple is lower than the crease under your breasts, then implants will not be very effective for you—your breasts droop too much and an implant will only exacerbate this. If you're unhappy with the appearance of your breasts and your nipple falls below the crease line, you might find satisfaction in a breast reduction, which, depending on the shape of the breasts, can be done in concert with an implant. Read Chapter 15, "Making Molehills out of Mountains: Breast Reduction," for more on breast reduction.

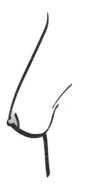

The nipple on this breast falls well below the crease. This breast is not a good candidate for breast implant surgery.

Sizing Up Your Breast Implant Options

OK, so you know you're not alone in your desire for larger or shapelier breasts, and while you might not want to end up in a size DD cup, you definitely want to move farther down the breast-cup alphabet. It's time, then, to take a closer look at the surgical options that are available to you. Breast-implant surgery is just what it sounds like—doctors surgically place a substance (silicone gel or saline filled implant) in the breast in order to change the shape of the breast and increase its size.

Cosmetic surgeons have been performing breast-implant surgery for decades, and even though there were often negative side effects, women were willing to put up with them in order to have the larger bust size they desired. Implants today have greatly improved, and testing and federal regulations abound in order to ensure that the implant your physician gives you will be as safe as possible.

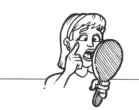

Wrinkle Ahead!

Over the years, doctors have used a variety of different substances for breast enlargement, including hand-carved sponges, human fat, liquid silicone, and silicone gel. Today, the only implant that is allowed by the Food and Drug Administration for new patients is a saline implant. If any cosmetic surgeon recommends anything else, be sure to get a second opinion!

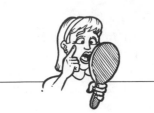

Wrinkle Ahead!

Under 18 years of age? Then it's illegal for you to get breast implants in some states. Check with your local medical board to find out what the law is in your state!

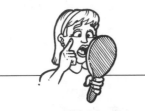

Wrinkle Ahead!

Some of the adverse side effects of liquid silicone injections (which are illegal) include lumpy breasts, and hard breasts. The hard lumps make it difficult to diagnose cancer, because doctors can't distinguish a tumor from a lump.

What an implant looks like.

Implant Materials

Here's a brief description about the various kinds of implants you'll probably hear about:

➤ **Saline implants.** Saline implants are the most common type of breast implant available today. As a matter of fact, unless you meet the criteria outlined in the section on silicone implants, saline implants are the only kind of implant that you can legally obtain in the United States. Saline implants have a silicone shell similar to that of the gel implant, but after the shell is placed in the breast, it is filled with saline (instead of silicone).

➤ **Liquid Silicone injections.** All forms of liquid silicone injections are illegal, and if your cosmetic surgeon ever suggests injecting liquid silicone in your breast, you should report him or her to the appropriate medical board.

➤ **Silicone Gel Implants.** Silicone gel implants have a solid silicone shell and are filled with a tightly knit silicone gel. The FDA restricted the use of silicone gel implants in 1992. Only people who have had gel implants before or meet special qualifications outlined below can have a gel implant. There have been no cases to date that prove a link between silicone and any disease.

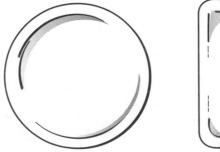
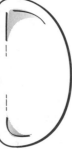

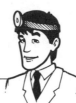

The Doctors Are In

Only breasts that meet the following criteria qualify for silicone gel implants:

➤ Rippling of an implant that shows or thin breast tissue

➤ Thin tissue cover

➤ A capsule (firming of the breast due to scar tissue formed around the implant) that would respond to a textured implant

➤ Had gel implants before and there is service required related to the implant, or the implant is not a problem but old enough to change out as preventative maintenance

Silicone gel implants look and feel better than saline implants, but until the regulations are changed, most women who want breast implants have no choice but to go with the saline implants.

Implant Texture

Implants are available with smooth or textured surfaces. Although you will not be able to feel the difference after the implant is placed in your breast, the texture can affect the long-term results.

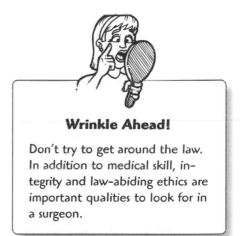

Wrinkle Ahead!

Don't try to get around the law. In addition to medical skill, integrity and law-abiding ethics are important qualities to look for in a surgeon.

➤ Textured implants are less likely to result in hard breasts because the texture prevents a capsule of your own tissue from forming around the implant.

➤ Textured implants tend to stay in position better, though there is some evidence that they contribute to breast rippling (read on for more about rippling).

➤ Smooth implants have a lower risk of breast rippling, although they are more likely to be displaced than textured implants.

159

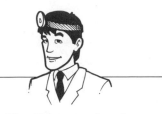

Risks Involved with Implants

Even though we believe the media blew the problems associated with silicone gel implants way out of proportion, that doesn't mean that breast implants are risk free. Read on to find out about the potential problems and side effects associated with breast-implant surgery;

➤ **Firming of the Breasts:** One of the most common problems associated with breast implants is overly firm breasts, which are caused by hard capsules forming around the implant (called "capsular contracture"). With the advancement of MRI studies and x-ray screenings (mammography), cancer can be detected if capsules begin to form around the implant.

➤ **Loss of Nipple Sensation:** There is a small chance that you will permanently lose your nipple sensation after implant surgery due to nerve damage during your surgery.

➤ **Implant Displacement:** The larger the implant, the more likely it will be displaced. Textured implants can help reduce the likelihood of displacement, but if an implant is displaced it can make the breasts look asymmetrical and shift the nipple in undesirable positions.

➤ **Implant Deflation:** Saline implants can leak and deflate. It's not dangerous, but the implant will need to be surgically removed and replaced.

➤ **Breast Rippling:** If this occurs, your saline implant can be exchanged for a textured gel implant. If your surgeon overfills the implant (which is safe), it might prevent rippling as well.

Eyes on the Size

Choosing the size of the implant can be the most difficult of the many decisions you'll need to make for breast implant surgery. Make sure you discuss the implant size with your doctor, and it is extremely important that you be honest with your doctor about your goals. He or she will not know what size breasts you want unless you are honest.

Implants come in a variety of sizes, with the most common ranging between 200 and 600 ml. As noted above, the larger the implant, the more likely it is to be displaced after surgery.

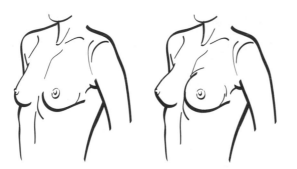

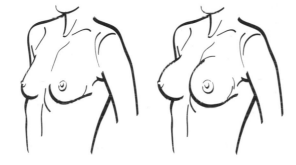

The small-breasted woman had a relatively small-sized implant (200 ml). The breasts are noticeably larger, but the breasts are still in proportion with the rest of her body.

Before and after pictures of someone who received a large (500 ml) implant.

Repeat Customers

It is essential that you are aware that breast-implant surgery typically does not last a patient's lifetime and will need to be repeated at least once.

Implant Positions and Breast Incisions

Although you don't have many choices when it comes to the kind of breast implant you can have, you might find yourself overwhelmed by the number of ways your implants can be inserted into your breasts. You'll want to discuss in minute detail with your doctor not only where the implant will be placed in your breast, but also where the incisions will be made in order to place the implants. The choices of implant location and the type of incisions your doctor makes are important because:

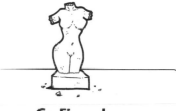

Go Figure!

A runway model who is 5'8" might tolerate a 300 cc implant. At 375 cc, unless you are very large or very tall, you are entering industrial-size range. If you get an implant that big, you might find it hard to make eye contact with a man again!

161

➤ Where your implant is placed will determine how your breasts look and feel.

➤ Where your doctor makes the incisions during surgery will dictate the kind of scar you will be left with.

➤ Some incisions are more detectable than others.

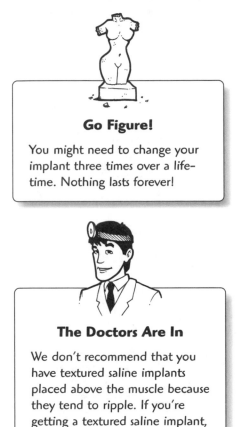

Go Figure!

You might need to change your implant three times over a lifetime. Nothing lasts forever!

The Doctors Are In

We don't recommend that you have textured saline implants placed above the muscle because they tend to ripple. If you're getting a textured saline implant, have it placed under the muscle.

We'll try to make the decision process easier by outlining the most common implant surgeries and telling you the pros and cons of each one.

Where Will Your Implant Rest in Your Breast?

Your breast consists mainly of skin, muscle, and glands. Implants can be inserted between different layers, and where they are placed affects how your breasts look and how well the implants last over time.

➤ **Placement of the implant above the muscle and under the gland.** This ages well as your breasts slip a little bit over the years with time and pregnancy. It also gives better cleavage.

➤ **Placement of the implant under the muscle.** Placement under the muscle, or submuscular placement, leads to a higher riding breast because the implants are positioned higher than where the breast will eventually rest (over time) and the implants don't droop with age. But that doesn't stop your breast from drooping eventually, and might cause your breasts to look a little higher and farther apart, too.

Incision Decisions

Cosmetic surgeons have found some very creative ways for inserting breast implants. Some of the ways make it very difficult to detect that a woman has had implant surgery; other ways are more quick-healing or make touch-up or replacement surgery easier. You'll want to discuss the following options with your cosmetic surgeon:

➤ **Incision placement at the edge of the nipple.** This incision allows easy reentry for touch-ups and replacement surgeries. There is a chance that your scars will show and your surgery will be detectable.

➤ **Incision placement at the center of the nipple.** The nipple heals well with this incision. We prefer the central-nipple procedure over the incision at the edge of the nipple because it is farther from the nerves. You decrease your chances of nerve damage from happening during surgery with this procedure.

➤ **Incision placement under the breast in the crease.** This incision placement can show in some cases, depending on how your breast rests. Talk with your surgeon about whether or not this incision placement will adequately conceal your scars.

➤ **Incisions under the armpit.** These incisions show only when you lift your arms, but it will be difficult for your doctor to reaccess these sites if follow-up surgeries are needed.

➤ **Belly-button incisions.** These incisions can be done for saline implants. Like armpit incisions, it will be difficult for your doctor to replace or touch up your surgery through the same incision later.

> **The Doctors Are In**
>
> One of the biggest concerns about silicone breast implants over the years has been whether they cause cancer. After research and formal studies, it was concluded that silicone implants certainly did not cause cancer, and that women with breast implants actually seemed to have fewer incidences of cancer than their unaugmented counterparts.

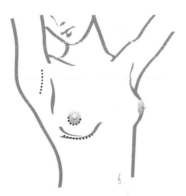

Where incisions can be made for implant surgery.

Since breast-implant surgery will probably need to be repeated, we recommend that you get incisions that are close to or on the breast, as it allows easier access. It is harder to remove an implant the farther it is from the incision site. You can't trade a saline for a gel implant through a belly-button incision and it is harder to do from the armpit.

When choosing implant and incision placement, it is important to take into account the kind of breast you have, your lifestyle, and how secret you want your surgery to be. Be sure to have a thorough discussion with your cosmetic surgeon to determine which surgery option is right for you!

Busting Out the Bucks

Given the pleasure that breast-enhancement surgery gives to women, the cost seems very reasonable to most women who have the procedure performed. Here is how the costs generally break down:

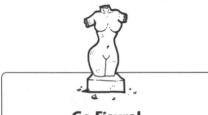

➤ **Facility fees.** Approximately $1,500 for surgery in an ambulatory center.

➤ **Anesthesiologist fees.** The fees will typically be $500–$600 unless the operation takes longer than normal.

➤ **Implants.** A pair of saline implants cost about $900 and a pair of gel implants is approximately $1,850.

➤ **Total fee.** Your total fee, including the doctor's fee, will be around $5,500 for saline implants and $7,200 for gel implants.

Go Figure!

The going rate in Beverly Hills is about $5,500 for saline implants and about $7,500 to replace implants with gels if the patient qualifies for them.

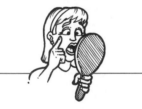

Wrinkle Ahead!

When considering the cost of breast implants, it is important to keep in mind that you will likely need to have touch-up or re-placement surgery, so you should be prepared to keep paying for your breasts into the future. If you're not financially able to cover the additional expenses, you should rethink having the surgery in the first place.

Free Sample?

Don't you wish it was possible to get a free sample of breast-implant surgery—just to see if it's right for you? Unfortunately, you can't. But you can try wearing a padded bra to see if you like how bigger breasts look on you. If you like the look, then you'll probably like the real thing, too!

Breast-Implant Checklist

Here are a few more things to keep in mind when you talk to your surgeon about breast-implant surgery:

➤ Make sure that you see the same type of implant that you are going to get and that you see it in the same condition that it will be when implanted into your body. Know the manufacturer, size, and price of your implant.

➤ The choice is yours to make as far as the placement of the incision.

➤ Discuss your anesthesia options with your surgeon. You can choose between general anesthesia or local anesthesia with sedation.

After Your Surgery

Plan to rest quietly after surgery and to sleep alone—it tends to prevent capsule formation. Your breasts will be swollen for two weeks to a month. Don't overexert yourself for several weeks, and don't resume strenuous activities that involve your breasts, such as sex or exercise, without your doctor's approval.

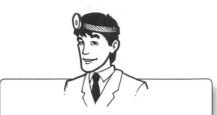

The Doctors Are In

Plan to have general anesthesia for secondary implant surgery. Scar tissue does not allow the spread of local anesthesia, and injecting local anesthesia can endanger the implant already in place.

When Your Cup Overflows

Whenyou go for augmentation, keep in mind that most women love their results. It is a safe surgery with an extremely high success rate. If you decide that breast augmentation is right for you, we think you'll enjoy your bigger, shapelier results!

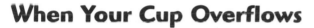

The Least You Need to Know

➤ Check with a doctor to find out if implants are right for you.

➤ Decide where you want your implants to be placed and where you want your incisions to be. Discuss this with your doctor and get his or her opinion. Ask for an explanation and any other questions you may have.

➤ Expect to have at least one touch-up surgery or replacement in your lifetime, and possibly as many as three.

➤ Remember, it's your body. You make all the decisions.

Chapter 15

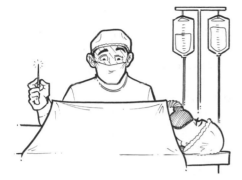

Making Molehills out of Mountains: Breast Reduction

In This Chapter

➤ When breasts are too large to handle

➤ Finding out if you're a good candidate for a breast reduction

➤ Looking over your breast-reduction options

➤ Breast-reduction techniques for men

➤ What to expect after your surgery

Big breasts aren't always a blessing, and they sometimes can cause problems that smaller-breasted women never imagine. Women often seek breast-reduction surgery in order to make their breasts look more attractive, to avoid loss of sensation due to stretched nerves, to alleviate back pain, and sometimes just to lighten the load!

If you're a man with excess breast tissue, then you might want to skip to the last section of this chapter, where we discuss what breast-reduction options are available to you.

Sizing Up Large Breasts

Not all large breasts need to be reduced, and some smaller breasts are good candidates for some of the procedures discussed in this chapter because of excessive drooping. Whether you have mild droop or your breasts practically reach your belly button, read on to find out what you can do to perk yourself up!

Fortunately, doctors have devoted years to developing breast-reduction techniques that look good and feel great.

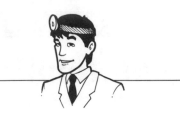

The Doctors Are In

Do not ask for breast reduction if you want to change the shape of your breasts. Breast reduction primarily reduces the *size* of your breasts. Implants change the *shape* of your breasts. Be clear to your cosmetic surgeon about what you're looking for.

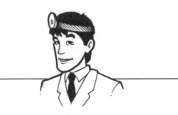

The Doctors Are In

If you are a candidate for breast-reduction surgery, electing to have early treatment will reduce the need for the more radical T-incision technique to be performed or the need to have extensive surgery later that can leave more noticeable scars.

Exchanging Old Breasts for New

Many breast lifts involve removing the excess skin that has stretched and causes the breast to droop. After the skin is removed and the skin is reattached, the breast will not droop as much and will rest in a higher position. There are some breast reductions that have almost undetectable scars or remove skin that are based on liposuction. Talk to your doctor about his or her individual technique for performing this kind of an operation.

There are a number of procedures available for women who want smaller breasts. Each procedure produces different scars and is effective for a particular condition. You should discuss the options with your cosmetic surgeon.

T-Incision Technique

The T-incision technique is a fairly radical procedure intended for women who have very large, misshapen breasts. In this procedure, an upside down T-shaped incision is made on the breast, which raises the nipple. The T incision today is usually very short and leaves a subtle scar.

Some large, misshapen breasts that have undergone this procedure will also need to be treated with implants in order to regain a natural shape and appearance. See Chapter 14, "Busting Up! Breast Augmentation," for information on breast implants.

The horizontal part of the T-shaped incision can show in your cleavage area, and when the nipple is raised the scar around the nipple shows.

The Vertical-Incision Lift

The vertical-incision lift is a viable alternative for women who want to have a breast reduced.

This is an excellent technique for small, droopy breasts and can sometimes be used to successfully reduce moderately large breasts. Very large breasts can respond favorably to this technique, but it is usually reserved only for smaller breasts that need to be surgically augmented because it takes the least amount of tissue out of the breast.

The Doughnut Lift

The doughnut-lift technique is usually used to alter the shape of smaller, droopy breasts that need to be augmented; however, some patients have had favorable results with this technique as a breast-reduction surgery. However, many have had extreme scars and stretching at the nipples.

Surgeons who perform this technique cut around the nipple and remove skin and sometimes breast tissue.

The doughnut lift is performed by making an incision around the nipple and another incision in the breast to remove skin and alleviate pressure on the breast. A scar can form and the nipple can stretch. The risks far out way the benefits and you can get better results with liposuction when it comes to achieving higher and firmer breasts.

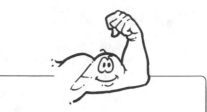

Better Definition

Mastoplexy is the catch-all term for breast-lifts that do not reduce size. They result in more attractive looking breasts. Suctioning the breast also gives ligaments relief from the weight of the breast and helps them to maintain their shape longer by reducing volume and weight.

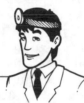

The Doctors Are In

Sometimes very young girls grow just one or both breasts to an overly large size. This is a condition called "virginal hypertrophy." It is a rare type of deformity that really can emotionally damage a developing young girl's personality. It is often a condition that can appear to look just like a tumor, and tumors need to be ruled out by your physician before a young woman can be adequately diagnosed. Virginal hypertrophy is not related to weight gain, and many of these girls that suffer from this condition are quite thin.

It's important to note that the doughnut lift can have very undesirable results, and you should avoid this procedure altogether or consider all other options before undergoing the procedure. Two significant risks are that both the nipple and the scar can spread to become extremely wide. When this occurs, it is very difficult to surgically repair—in some cases, impossible. If you are contemplating having this technique performed to reduce your breast size, consider the risks before you decide whether or not to move ahead with this surgery.

The Suction Lift

One of our favorite techniques for breast reduction today is the suction lift. Many women have found this technique to be very effective and highly successful in reducing breast size and leaving a natural and attractive appearance. It is performed by having one or two incision sites made, suctioning out tissue and fat, and closing the incisions so that they are difficult to detect if you heal well. When the problem of overly developed breasts first begins, this technique (if performed early) can be a ligament-sparing and skin-sparing procedure.

It allows you to reduce the weight and shape of your breasts because your doctor can remove unwanted fat and breast tissue before they stretch your breasts out of shape and cause a major loss of skin elasticity. This is suitable surgery for young women and might protect them from later damage of overly developed breasts.

Suction seems to be the least invasive method with the least amount of scarring. It tends to preserve vessels, nerves, and the supportive ligaments in the breast.

Suction and Quadrant Trimming

There is a new technique available that Dr. Semel created that combines breast suctioning and quadrant trimming of the breast from the inside. In other words, one or two incisions are made, suction is performed, and then the incision sites are closed. The incision sites are strategically placed to avoid obvious detection and are usually well hidden when you heal in an ideal fashion. A splint must be worn on the breast for three weeks to help guide the breast into its new form. Otherwise the skin of the breast may not attach well to its newly created mound (underlying structure).

It carries the same risks of any breast reduction, including skin or nipple loss, change or loss of sensation, and loss of ability to lactate.

Two different breast-reduction procedures. The dashed lines represent the incisions.

Implants and Breast Lifts

It will probably be necessary to get a breast implant along with a reduction when the breasts have emptied or all the breast tissue hangs below where it needs to be. Your doctor can sew breast tissue up high but, unfortunately, it won't stay long-term without the use of an implant. In any of the procedures we've mentioned, an implant can be placed and the tissue can be trimmed around the implant to accommodate it. This provides you with higher-resting breast tissue and cleavage that usually cannot be obtained with just the use of your own breast tissue. See Chapter 14, "Busting Up! Breast Augmentation" for more information about breast implants.

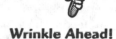

Wrinkle Ahead!

Risks of breast surgery include bleeding, loss of sensation, nerve damage, scarring, infection, skin loss, nipple loss, loss of lactation, and recurrence (regrowth of breast tissue for women who have reduction).

We suggest that you consider all of the breast-reduction techniques that are currently available and discuss with your surgeon which surgical alternative might best meet your cosmetic needs.

For Men Only

Let's face it: Big breasts on men is an undesirable characteristic. Large breasts on men can develop from congenital conditions or from taking muscle-building drugs (anabolic steroids) that are illegal now in the United States. In the congenital cases or the steroid cases, a *fibroadenoma* forms which is firm and lumpy and is usually not cancer in 99 percent of cases.

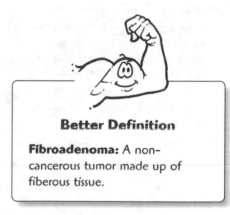

Better Definition

Fibroadenoma: A non-cancerous tumor made up of fiberous tissue.

Typically, a small semicircular incision has to be made in the center of the breast by a surgeon, just as is done in women. The fibroma is teased out along with excess fat. This can be done through a 5–7 millimeter incision in the center of the breast.

No matter how big the breasts have become in men, the skin almost always contracts after the fibroma is removed.

If you think that you may suffer from this condition, consult with your physician at once and have him or her talk you through the operation step by step!

Letting It All Hang Out

Not everyone should have their breasts reduced. It is a wonderful surgery that produces amazing results, but some women don't need a reduction, some women just need an implant, and some women don't need anything! Some women need mildly intervening liposuction, while others need a great deal of surgery. The more surgery you need to have performed, the more risk there is involved. Of course, it would be better if you didn't need to have any surgery performed, but you might just be one of the women who are a candidate for this surgery. Our following suggestions should help you to decide what options best fit your needs:

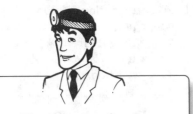

The Doctors Are In

Bring a bra that you would like to look great in to communicate your desired size, or show the doctor photos of what you're hoping to achieve. Talk to your doctor about everything that concerns you about your breasts. He or she cannot read your mind.

➤ Strongly consider suction if your nipple is higher than the crease under your breast.

➤ If your nipple is at, but not lower than, the crease under your breast, you need a reduction or a mastoplexy with or without an implant.

➤ When your nipple is below the crease of your breast, you need reduction surgery.

➤ If you are overweight, try to lose weight before you have your breast-reduction surgery performed. Anticipate that everything will be a different size and in a new position after you lose weight.

➤ Do not have reduction surgery if you ever plan to nurse a baby. It is currently unknown whether suction will have an effect on lactation.

➤ Do not have reduction surgery if you plan to get pregnant very soon.

➤ Plan on more than one surgery with more scarring than usual if your breasts are very large.

Consider all of the breast-reduction techniques that we have discussed. Think about the results and the risks of each surgery. Then, choose a surgery that you are the best candidate for. Next, schedule an appointment with your cosmetic surgeon to discuss your breast-reduction needs. Be sure to ask his or her opinion about your condition and discuss which breast-reduction alternative he or she thinks would best meet your cosmetic needs.

Costs

If you are a woman, expect to pay between $8,000 and $8,500 for breast reduction surgery. Breast-reduction surgery for men typically costs around $5,000.

Lightening Your Load

There are certain rules that apply to all surgery, including the following:

➤ Get a physical.

➤ Go on a high-protein diet.

➤ Take lots of minerals and vitamins.

➤ Stay off anticoagulants two weeks prior to surgery.

➤ Lose weight or be weight stable if your surgery involves liposuction or any kind or reduction surgery.

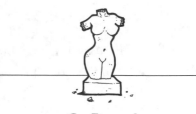

Go Figure!

No two breasts are ever exactly alike. Surgery might make your breasts look more alike, but don't expect it to make them identical.

The New, Smaller-Breasted You!

Breast reduction is an easier surgery to recover from than it is to plan for. When all goes well, you should not have much postoperative pain. We suggest that you be as quiet as possible and follow our postoperative tips listed below for a speedy recovery:

➤ Take Arnica to help control bruising until it goes away. Arnica is a bruise-reducing herb that you can find at your local health food store. It helps if you start before the surgery.

➤ Keep your dressings dry. Your doctor may allow you to trade them for a bra in a few days.

➤ Activity will spread your scars and can pull the surgery apart. We recommend a quiet and predominantly sedentary recovery period, but you do not have to be in bed all the time. It's important to do some walking because remaining completely inactive can cause blood clots to develop.

➤ Ice your breasts the first few days. It will reduce swelling.

➤ Don't take pain pills if you don't hurt.

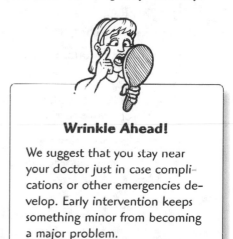

Wrinkle Ahead!

We suggest that you stay near your doctor just in case complications or other emergencies develop. Early intervention keeps something minor from becoming a major problem.

➤ Take your antibiotics. Surgery is one of the times you need them the most to fight off infection. This is especially important if you have had implants inserted. Without antibiotics, your body may reject your implants!

➤ Don't fly for 12 to 14 days after surgery.

Keep in mind that the techniques for breast reduction have improved to the point that people with small problems can have a small amount of surgery to correct them and be back to work with relatively little downtime. It can be an easy recovery for most people. If your job does not require you to perform manual labor, you can return to work in just a few short weeks.

The results are long lasting, although touch-up surgeries might be required and implants might have to be replaced once or twice in your lifetime.

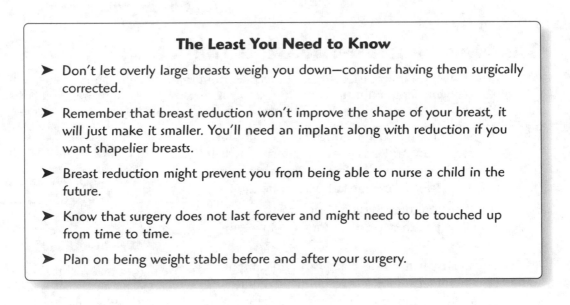

The Least You Need to Know

➤ Don't let overly large breasts weigh you down—consider having them surgically corrected.

➤ Remember that breast reduction won't improve the shape of your breast, it will just make it smaller. You'll need an implant along with reduction if you want shapelier breasts.

➤ Breast reduction might prevent you from being able to nurse a child in the future.

➤ Know that surgery does not last forever and might need to be touched up from time to time.

➤ Plan on being weight stable before and after your surgery.

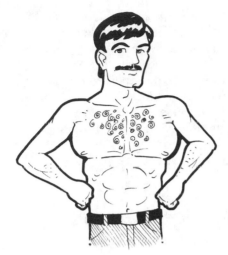

Chapter 16

For Men Only: Pectoral Implants

> ## In This Chapter
>
> ➤ What's available for men who desire bigger chests
>
> ➤ How pectoral implants are surgically placed
>
> ➤ Considering the side effects of pectoral implants
>
> ➤ Other options for increasing the size of your chest
>
> ➤ What you can do to prepare for and recover from your procedure

Muscle enlargement and greater chest definition are common goals for many athletic-minded men. These goals are difficult to achieve through exercise and take much longer to accomplish at the gym than they do in the operating room. For men who are willing to trade the actual development of their pectoral muscles for the appearance of these muscles and greater definition, pectoral implants are available today that can produce these desired results.

Rising to the Occasion: Who Can Benefit from Pectoral Implants?

Most men do not need pectoral-implantation surgery, but some men want the surgery performed. It is important to such men to look their best, and they either want chest implants to improve a physical deficit due to a deformity caused by illness or to enhance the size of the pectoral muscles that they have already developed at the gym.

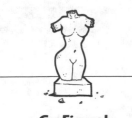

Go Figure!

The pectoral is one of the fastest-growing muscles and often grows in proportion with arm musculature. In some cases, though, pectoral muscles do not respond to exercise because the muscles do not fire. If you discover that you have muscles that do not fire, electrical stimulation of the muscles should be attempted, followed by exercise, to see if coordinated firing of all the muscle fibers can be achieved. If that's unsuccessful, then you might want to consider pectoral implants.

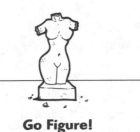

Go Figure!

Although pectoral implants are performed, they are not done in any significant number yearly in the United States. They are usually performed on men with body-builder shapes or those who are significantly underdeveloped in the pectoral area.

Others who elect to have this surgery have tried to improve their pectoral size through exercise but have not achieved maximum results or are unable to exercise for medical reasons and would like a little cosmetic improvement. Another group of men who seek this surgery are those who have suffered tendon tearing of the pectoral muscle that has caused one pectoral muscle to remain smaller in size than the other one. All of these men are candidates for pectoral-implantation surgery and might benefit from this highly successful surgery.

Anabolic Steroids and Your Health

Some men take matters into their own hands and have resorted to illegal anabolic steroid use in order to develop larger pectoral muscles. Unrestricted and unsupervised use of steroids can cause severe liver and heart problems over a long period of time and limit your life expectancy. When steroids are discontinued, the muscles tend to atrophy and return to near or at their original size (if the results are not maintained through massive calorie intake and excessive exercise).

If you are a young man who is not finished growing and you take steroids, you will permanently stunt your own growth. Anabolic steroids close the growth center in the bones and cause long bones to stop advancing, and growth is permanently stunted. Consider these adverse effects and ask yourself if these harmful effects are a price you would be willing to pay for larger pectorals. We recommend that this illegal alternative be avoided at all costs.

Perking Up!

The most up-to-date technique for improving your pectoral muscles is chest-implantation surgery. Pectoral implants come in custom sizes to measure and common stock sizes. If you are lucky, one of the standard sizes that are made in large volume—and are cheaper than the custom sizes—will fit you. The sizes come in small, medium, and large, just like breasts implants did when they were first manufactured. If there is not an appropriate size available for you, you can have one custom-made or your surgeon can trim an implant to fit your exact chest muscle. You'll want to consult with your surgeon about the size that is most appropriate for you.

The Surgical Procedure

During your chest-implant surgery, an incision will be made in your armpit. The implant will be folded and rotated into a pocket that will be surgically opened under your pectoral muscles. It is important that the implant you choose for your surgery is short enough so that it will not move toward your armpit, where the main vessels and nerves that are responsible for your arm and hand movement are located. If your implant is positioned too closely to this area, it could shift and injure these vessels and nerves. This could have a debilitating or even a deadly effect on you. For this reason, be sure that your surgeon specializes in chest-implantation surgery, has performed many of these operations, and assists you in choosing a properly sized implant. Most surgeons have not performed many of these surgeries, so be sure to choose one who has.

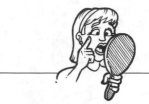

Wrinkle Ahead!

Anabolic steroids are available by prescription only because unsupervised use can have adverse side effects on a man's health. They are available by prescription for cancer and AIDS sufferers. Anabolic steroid use for athletic use is illegal.

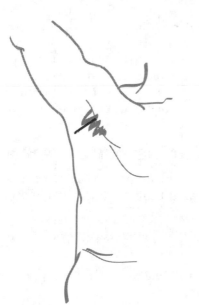

The incision for inserting the implant. It will be made under both arms.

The dashed line represents the position of the implant. It will be placed under the pectoral muscle.

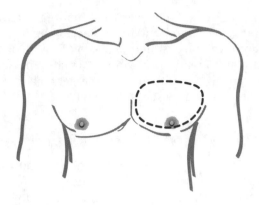

Making an Informed Decision

This is not a surgery to sign up for without carefully considering all of the facts. The risks of this operation must be weighed carefully. Your pectoral implants must be

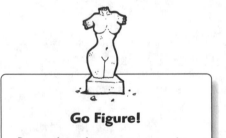

Go Figure!

Pectoral-implant surgery requires general anesthesia, which will relax your muscles and keep you pain-free during your surgery.

placed safely away from main vessels and nerves in the arms or else they can cause damage or death. The implants might also form capsules (tissue around the implant), become very firm, and grow slightly round. These last three results are rare, but they can occur.

Also, don't be surprised if you or others can feel the implant in place. The implants do not create the exact definition of well-exercised pectorals and become round in appearance over time. They do not move as you move when you raise your arms. They are detectable to a trained eye, but those in who are not in the know may not notice unless they feel them or notice that your pectorals are overly round.

Getting Big Ideas: Preparing for Surgery

The most important thing about preparing for pectoral-implant surgery is thorough investigation. Some of the most important things you should know about the effects of this surgery are:

➤ There will be underarm scars and the implants will give you some increased shape and size.

➤ If your implants are large, they will tend to show when you elevate your arms and at the top sides of your chest.

➤ You might need to have replacement surgery during your lifetime. The surgery is too new to determine if it will be needed and how often.

178

➤ Pectoral muscle implants have a particular look that is different from a look that is created at the gym. The definition between the muscles is not increased, and the bulk of the muscle is not as close as it would be if developed at the gym or by a combination of electrical stimulation and the gym.

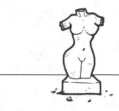

Go Figure!

If you cannot exercise for any medical reason, it is better to have something than nothing. Go for an implant! In an open shirt, jacket, or T-shirt, chest implants can look great!

How Much for Those Pecs?

Pectoral implant surgery will generally cost around $7,200, including the surgeon's fee, the anesthesiologist's fee, and operating room costs.

Preoperative Tips

Consider these preoperative tips before you decide this surgery is the one for you:

➤ Avoid anticoagulants and other performance-enhancing medications.

➤ Don't pump up or irritate your pectoral muscles for several weeks before the surgery.

➤ Arrange for aftercare and a driver. Your motion will be limited and the postoperative period can be painful, and you will need to use your pain medications. You will need a friend or nurse for a few days to look after you and get you around.

➤ Prepare ice in some quantity for your chest: It will control pain and swelling in the first two days and limit your need for pain pills.

➤ Reaching for anything can easily unseat or move your implant in the days following surgery.

➤ Be sure you are in good shape. General anesthesia is desirable for this one! That means clean lungs and a clean cardiovascular system—no smoking and lots of aerobic exercise the few weeks prior to your operation.

Keep these facts and tips in mind. Review our suggestions before signing up for this operation. Your appearance and mobility after surgery will count on them!

Inflating Those Pecs

If you've decided that this surgery is for you, then you're on your way from deflation to elation. Barring any complications, most men are very satisfied with the long-lasting results of this operation. It can take you from deflation to elation in just under an hour, and your implants will probably only need to be replaced once in your lifetime. Once your surgery has been performed, consider our postoperative tips:

➤ This is a tender procedure and you will need your pain pills and sleeping medication.

➤ You need to be meticulous about your antibiotics and vigilant about the possibility of contaminating your wounds with exposure to your house pets.

➤ You need to limit arm motion. Activity can precipitate a cramp in the overlying pectoral muscles that are already stretched.

➤ You need to be able to sleep. Clear your schedule.

➤ Be sure you and your doctor choose an implant that is the appropriate size so that is as close to proper proportion with your arms as possible.

➤ You need a helper for the first four or five days or so because you can't drive or do too much for yourself.

➤ You must keep the incisions dry. No showers!

➤ You will also notice that your chest muscles will be sore and swollen. It might take up to 12 weeks until you can consider working out at the gym again or performing other activities that require strenuous movement.

➤ It will be very difficult for you to move your arms at first.

All of these conditions are normal and will subside in time. Our pre- and postoperative tips in this chapter will help you to prepare and effectively deal with all of the effects of your pectoral-implant surgery.

Oh, and we forgot one more postoperative tip: Once you've recovered from your surgery, stock up on tank tops and show off that chest!

The Least You Need to Know

➤ Don't get pectoral implants unless you've tried other ways to increase your chest size.

➤ Be prepared to have pectoral implants replaced at least once your lifetime.

➤ Never take anabolic steroids to increase the size of your chest.

Part 4

Awesome Abdomens and Buttocks

Tummy tucks, midsection improvements, and fanny tucks are distinctly different from most cosmetic operations because they all require liposuction. Liposuction comes with its own preoperative and postoperative requirements that you'll need to be aware of before making a fully informed decision. The good news is that the additional requirements are usually rewarded with outstanding results!

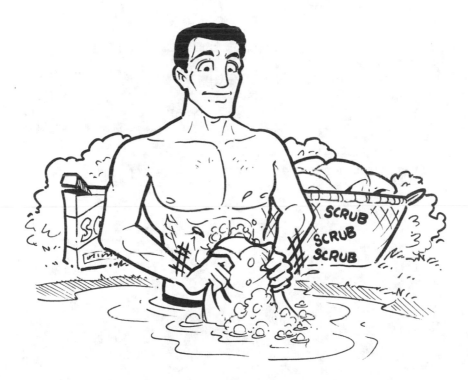

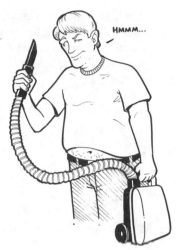

HMMM...

Chapter 17

Meeting in the Middle: Liposuction of the Midsection

In This Chapter

➤ Understanding what liposuction can do for your midsection

➤ Finding out if you're a good candidate for liposuction

➤ Preparing for and recovering from liposuction surgery

➤ A few words about abdominoplasty

➤ Considering the costs

Can you pinch an inch? If so, one solution to those love handles might just be liposuction. While liposuction should not be the first line of defense against tummy, side, and back fat, it is a popular surgery that can provide good results.

This Thing Called "Liposuction"

Liposuction is the most popular cosmetic procedure performed in the United States today. Cosmetic surgeons have been performing it for 20 years, and they have developed techniques that make it very effective for eliminating hard-to-lose fat.

We briefly discussed the liposuction procedure in Chapter 12, "Let's Neck! Neck Liposuction," but we'll review it again here as well.

Liposuction is typically performed via a few small incisions in the area where the fat will be removed. Before your surgeon actually sucks out your excess fat, he or she will inject a fluid into the area to be treated that will control bleeding, making it easier to suck out the fat. The doctor will then insert a narrow hollow rod that is attached to a suction machine or syringe and will suck out the fat. After your surgery, you will likely be asked to wear a liposuction garment, which is similar to a tight spandex girdle (leotards also work well), to aid in healing and skin contracture.

Spot Liposuction

Unless you have the body of a supermodel, spot liposuction is probably not the type of procedure you will need—unless it is for a touch-up. Spot liposuction is intended for removing small bits of fat that are resistant to diet or fat that comes back immediately after dieting. The small fatty spot is marked, an incision is made, the fat is suctioned so that it looks even with its surrounding areas, and then the incision is closed. Unfortunately, most of us need to remove more fat than spot liposuction is meant to remove.

Full-Circumference Liposuction

Full-circumference liposuction is a fairly new approach to liposuction that was developed to prevent a common problem associated with liposuction: If the fat isn't removed from an entire area, the area where the fat isn't removed tends to gain more fat. For example, if a patient's front abdomen is liposuctioned but not the back, fat is gained on the back; similarly, if the back is done, the front gains more fat. If the entire area is liposuctioned—front, back, and sides—then the fat is much less likely to come back.

Liposuctioning whole areas thoroughly will give you a better long-term result than focusing on only parts of an area, unless the patient only has small spots of fat.

Although incision placement varies from surgeon to surgeon, common incision sites for a full-circumference liposuction of the midsection are the belly button, pubic area, and the crease of the buttocks.

Incision placement for liposuction of the abdomen and back.

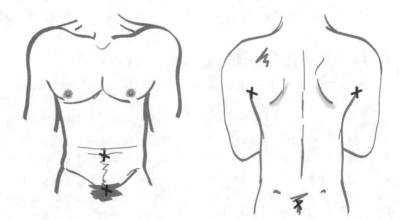

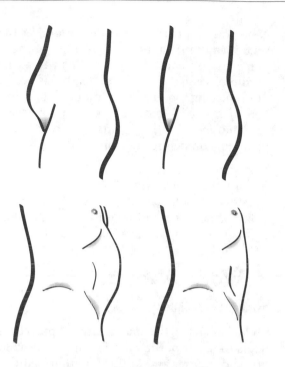

Before and after stomach liposuction on a female patient.

Before and after stomach liposuction on a male patient.

What to Watch Out For

It was understood quite early that removing too much fat made the skin stick too tight to the underlying structures. In other words, if too much fat was removed, you would end up looking weird! Not enough suction or suction to sculpt certain areas tended to become divots over time as the fat came back around the areas that were treated. When the skin did not drape correctly after surgery, it was usually because fat was left above the treated area and it sagged down, or fat from untreated areas simply grew around the treated sites, creating the illusion of divots.

When you choose a surgeon to perform your liposuction operation, ask to see pictures of your doctor's patients who have had the same surgery 12 months ago or longer. Be certain that they have not ended up with these kinds of results.

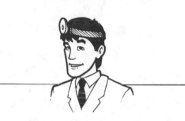

The Doctors Are In

Up to four pounds of fat can be removed without a blood transfusion. Surgery traumatizes blood vessels and red blood cells, protein disappears into the tissue, circulation is decreased, and the patient can become anemic. New blood can remedy this problem. Your own blood can and should be prepared in advance if greater than four pounds is required.

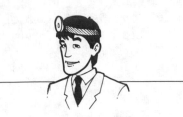

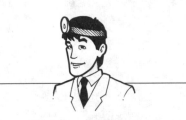

Nine pounds of fat is a safe amount of fat that can be suctioned during a liposuction surgery when blood is prepared. Any more than that puts you at high risk for fluid replacement problems. Death has been caused by not replacing blood or by too much fluid replacement. For the sake of a smooth surgery, antibiotics and after care that monitor fluid shifts should be discussed with your surgeon before your operation.

If you are generally overweight and the fat is not depot fat, liposuction will not help you. Liposuction does help people with depot fat who have dietary control. The depots are located in women at the arms and legs, and in men at the abdomen and back.

A Word About Abdominoplasty

Abdominoplasty is a major surgical procedure that refers to repair of the muscle wall of the abdomen and lifting or tightening of the abdominal skin, and it is not the best way to lose weight or reduce the amount of fat a patient has. When there are smaller problems of these areas, minor surgeries (like liposuction) can suit your cosmetic needs.

Abdominoplasty is not for everyone. The people who need it have abdominal skin that has lost its elasticity and have stretch marks. This can be from weight fluctuation, aging, pregnancy, or multiple childbirths that caused an increase in abdominal size. Large children, multiple births, and genetics are all factors that determine whether or not the abdominal muscles spread apart. The abdominal muscles can also be weakened from extensive or repeated abdominal surgery or accident or trauma (being punched too hard).

If you need an abdominoplasty, you want to be as thin as you can be before having it done. Some people with bad skin and good muscles want to have their abdominal girth trimmed. Abdominoplasty leaves scars which are usually unattractive and unsightly when nude. It has been used for chunky, really heavy people, but the fat comes back and the scars stretch and it really isn't used for this purpose anymore. Liposuction followed by a reasonable diet regimen protects better from this type of recurrence.

Qualifying for Liposuction ... and the Winner Is!

Not everyone qualifies for liposuction surgery; it takes more than just a desire for a trimmer stomach. Read on to find out about what makes someone a good candidate for liposuction:

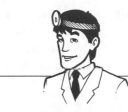

➤ **Lose weight before your surgery.** If you are considering liposuction, you obviously need to lose weight, right? So give yourself a head start on your liposuction surgery by losing the weight before your operation. It will help to get your body ready for the operation and can eventually assist you in maintaining your liposuction results.

> **The Doctors Are In**
>
> Liposuction is not a license to overeat. Fat cells in other parts of your body that have not been removed by liposuction can grow larger. Maintain a healthy diet even after your liposuction surgery.

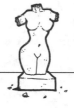

> **Go Figure!**
>
> Liposuction was first attempted in 1976 in Switzerland, without a good cosmetic result. It was performed with a "pluck-and-suck" approach, a lot like a plumbing machine. This early technique caused excessive ripping and tearing of blood vessels, tissue, and nerves. In addition, the skin did not contract after the fat was removed, so people were left with sagging skin. Too much fluid was also generated by disruption of the small blood vessels and underlying structures that were attached to the skin. This caused intense and agonizing swelling. Obviously, the surgery needed to be perfected!

➤ **Be weight stable for at least a few months.** If you have a tendency to gain and lose weight, be sure that you have achieved a weight that is realistic for you to maintain before your surgery. This will help ensure that your liposuction results will last for a long time and that you will not need to have the surgery repeated later on. Weight fluctuation can sometimes have an effect on the ultimate appearance of your liposuction results.

➤ **Avoid using liposuction as a replacement for healthy eating.** Liposuction can aid in removing unwanted fat, but it is no substitute for healthy eating or dieting, which are still two of the best ways to lose and maintain an attractive weight! Only use liposuction as a supplemental way of removing unwanted fat. It can be used in addition to healthy eating and dieting, but never as a replacement.

➤ **Exercise regularly.** One way to ensure that your liposuction results last is to develop a realistic exercise program that you can begin before your surgery and maintain afterward. Exercise will help to keep your weight stable and prevent any complications from developing after your liposuction. It is best to begin a regular exercise program before your operation so that you know that it is one you can stick to. Exercise regularly—your appearance relies on it!

➤ **Liposuction is not a cure for overeating.** We just can't say it enough! Liposuction is not a cure-all for consuming extra calories. We wouldn't want you to fool yourself into thinking that liposuction is an inexpensive and desirable way to consistently lose or maintain weight loss. The truth is, liposuction is expensive, and major liposuction surgeries that are repeated several times can be very taxing on your body. Be kind to your body and keep your liposuction surgeries to a minimum by not overeating.

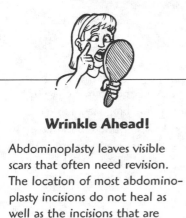

Wrinkle Ahead!

Abdominoplasty leaves visible scars that often need revision. The location of most abdominoplasty incisions do not heal as well as the incisions that are placed on other parts of the body for other surgeries.

➤ **Know your problem areas.** Understand which are your most resistant depot sites for weight loss. These are the sites that will need to be treated first. We suggest that you undress and take a realistic look at your body in a full-length mirror to determine which areas are the most troublesome for you. This will help you to get the results you want and prevent you from being talked into additional liposuction that you do not need or want.

Not for Obese People

Although liposuction removes fat, it is not well-suited for obese people. You must weigh over 20 percent of the average weight for your height and age to be considered obese. This surgery is not well suited for obese people because suctioning out a portion of fat from a body that is fraught with fat gives an abnormal-looking appearance. It is much better for an obese person to lose weight first, and then have a liposuction surgery performed. It results in a much more natural appearance.

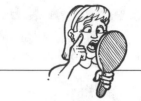

If you are confident that you can prepare yourself for surgery and maintain a healthy lifestyle after surgery, then make an appointment for a consult with your cosmetic surgeon. What've you got to lose … except a few pounds, of course!

Going the Liposuction Distance: Preop Tips

Once you have become a liposuction candidate, there are a few preoperative tips you should know. These tips will help you to get the best result from your operation and promote an uncomplicated recovery.

Give blood … to yourself!

You'll need to plan ahead and donate blood to yourself so it can be used during your surgery. Blood transfusions are often routine practice during a liposuction procedure, and it is best if your blood supply is replaced with its own blood rather than someone else's. You'll need to arrange to freeze your whole blood, not just the cells, at a reliable blood bank. After your surgery, your blood can be used if more than three pounds has been removed. You need a unit for each additional three to four pounds of fat that have been removed.

Take protein powder to give your body the necessary building blocks for surgery.

The protein will give your body the ability to heal your incisions that it needs to recover from surgery.

Take a multiple vitamin or vitamin powder.

Remember, your body will be working overtime to recover from surgery. It will need all the help it can get. Taking vitamins will help to give it the extra nutrients that it needs.

Wrinkle Ahead!

Liposuction surgery is different from face-lift operations, where patients can go in and have their operations touched up from time to time. Liposuction is an invasive procedure and should be performed in conjunction with dieting, not as a replacement for dieting. Liposuction results can be maintained with weight loss and dietary control.

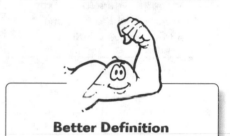

Better Definition

Obesity: Someone who is obese is over 20 percent of their ideal weight or the average weight of someone for their age, height, and bone structure.

Take Vitamin K before surgery.

This is a prescription medication. The vitamin helps the clotting process of the blood. The faster your blood clots, the faster you will heal!

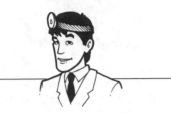

The Doctors Are In

Take B complex with folic acid and B12 with iron (325 micrograms) when you are preparing to give blood and before your surgery. It helps to absorb iron that you will need to produce blood cells for surgery or blood donation (to yourself). Ask your doctor about this option and about alternative solutions.

Get accustomed to a healthy diet and exercise.

Without a healthy diet and exercise, liposuction will fail over time. Liposuction surgery is not like a manicure or hair-coloring treatment: holding still for it is not enough, you need to exercise to maintain the results!

Consider all off these preoperative suggestions before you go in for liposuction surgery. You'll stay leaner longer if you follow these health tips.

How to Take Care of a Skinnier You: Postoperative Tips

Liposuction usually has a high success rate, but it can be painful to recover from. Once you've had your liposuction operation, there are things you can do to speed up your recovery and make it as comfortable as possible:

➤ When your fat depots have shrunk from dieting, you can treat the fat depots left after the liposuction while they are smaller and easier to suction. The less volume of fat there is to be suctioned, the less time and less blood is needed for surgery. You will also heal more easily.

➤ Never let your guard down—always watch your diet!

➤ Take all pain medication prescribed by your doctor.

➤ Avoid the sun and tanning beds. This can cause bruise marks to last longer or become permanent. It can also slow down the shrinkage or contraction of your skin.

➤ Wear a supportive garment with light pressure to help your skin contract over the postoperative months. Skin contraction can take time. Check out your local dance store for a leotard or lycra shirt or pants to wear.

➤ Take a dip! Warm baths and Jacuzzi sessions help skin to contract. It is unclear what exactly the water does, but it does appear to have some therapeutic effect on the skin. If a pool is available, swimming is also effective. Immersion for 20 minutes a day in water is a must; showers are not a substitute.

Take our advice and you'll probably end up looking fabulous!

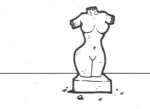

Go Figure!

Fat cells can grow larger. If you overeat after liposuction, they can grow so big that you can lose your new and improved appearance.

The Price of a Slimmer Midsection

The cost of full-circumference liposuction of the midsection varies according to how much fat needs to be removed, but you can expect to pay between $6,000 and $8,000, including doctor's fee and operating room costs, for the procedure.

If at First You Don't Succeed ...

When a liposuction result is uneven, fat transplants and selective additional reduction can be carried out. The most common problem that needs revision liposuction is asymmetric fat deposits, which doctors can correct via liposuction on the larger area. We encourage you to wait at least nine to twelve months before having a revision procedure in order to make sure that the problem is permanent (and thus needs to be revised)

Because fat cells are suctioned out during your liposuction procedure, the results of liposuction should be long-lasting. That is, if your weight remains stable! If you gain weight after you have a liposuction procedure, the remaining fat cells get bigger, putting you right back where you started (the remaining fat cells in other parts of your body will enlarge). It's very important that you are committed to being physically fit before you have liposuction, otherwise, the results will be fleeting.

The Least You Need to Know

➤ Typically you should plan to have a full-circumference liposuction.

➤ Lose weight and be weight stable before your liposuction surgery.

➤ Liposuction is not a license to overeat. Your remaining fat cells in surrounding areas can still grow larger.

➤ Liposuction is not a weight-loss solution for obese people.

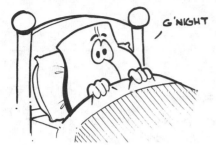

Chapter 18

G'NIGHT

Bringing Up the Rear: Fanny Tucks and Liposuction

> ## In This Chapter
>
> ➤ The role of diet and exercise in maintaining a firm and shapely fanny
>
> ➤ Creating a firm platform for your surgeon to build on
>
> ➤ Butt sculpting and other liposuction procedures
>
> ➤ How to prepare for and recover from your procedure

Got a little more fanny than you wish you had? Or maybe you're happy with the size of your rear, but perhaps it's droopy or otherwise misshapen. In this chapter we'll cover the surgical and nonsurgical options available to improve the shape and size of your buttocks.

Not Your Grandmother's Fanny Tuck!

The term "fanny tuck" continues to be used by many people today, but the surgery does not.

The treatments available today to reshape fannies are less invasive and more successful than old-fashioned fanny-tuck surgeries.

Bringing Up the Rear

If you take care of yourself with proper diet and exercise, you probably will not need to have any kind of cosmetic improvements made to your fanny. However, if these preventative measures are not enough to keep your fanny in shape, you might want to consider having your fanny cosmetically improved.

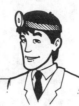

The Doctors Are In

Traditional fanny-tuck surgeries, in which large buttock mass is surgically extracted, tissue is lifted, and excess skin is removed, are still performed today under special circumstances (for example, if removal of the skin will reduce the appearance of a scar). The surgery is recommended only for those who want to fit and look better in their clothes, not for the person who wants to wear revealing clothes at the pool or a high-cut bathing suit at the beach.

Butt Sculpting

If your fanny is just beginning to lose its shape, you might think about fat transplants, or what is referred to as liposculpture. This procedure has replaced the traditional fanny tuck as the procedure of choice for misshapen buttocks. In a liposculpture procedure, the physician removes fat from one part of the body and transplants it to another part of the body (the fanny). This is done with a syringe and needle, not a knife. In some cases, there is a general reduction in size of the entire fatty mass of the buttocks, but often the fanny is simply reshaped.

Doctors typically remove fat from the inner thigh or lower part of the buttock and immediately transfer to the upper and outer buttock to make it ride higher and fuller, creating a more desirable shape. This is done on an as-needed basis, a little bit at a time. This causes little disability when a little is done at a time.

If you decide to have fat transplanted from one part of your body to your buttocks, make sure that the fat is not taken from your stomach, because stomach fat fluctuates too much and will probably be the first to go when you lose weight. Instead, ask your surgeon to take fat from a place like your thigh. Thigh fat is more stable or stubborn and is more difficult to lose than fat from other parts of your body. It is usually one of the last places that lose fat when you lose weight. Love handles (from your lower back) are also a great transplant choice.

Fanny tucks today do not have to create a larger butt. You can reposition the fat in your butt to create a rounder (but not necessarily a larger) butt.

Butt Liposuction

If you are satisfied with the shape (roundness) of your fanny but are dissatisfied with its size because you believe it is too big, then you will most likely benefit from liposuction. In order for liposuction to be effective, your skin must still have its elasticity. Liposuction can help to reduce fanny size while maintaining its round shape, but your results must be maintained through diet and exercise. For details of the liposuction procedure, refer to Chapter 17, "Meeting in the Middle: Liposuction of the Midsection."

In smaller patients, the fat that is in the lower part of the butt is usually suctioned by hand and transferred to the upper part of the buttock. In the case of very large patients, full liposuction that discards the excess fat can be carried out. When this is done, if more than four pounds is likely to be removed (2,000 cc), a unit or two of your whole blood should be available in order to return protein and cells after the surgery. When a large amount of fat is removed, sometimes the patient loses enough blood to warrant a blood transfusion. It is preferable to have your own blood available for a transfusion in case it is needed. Not all surgeons do this, so be sure that your surgeon does!

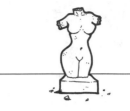

Go Figure!

Cosmetic surgeons recognize two styles of buttocks today: the Brazilian, with no crease beneath the buttocks, and the European, with a crease beneath the buttocks. The Brazilian style gives the advantage of fat below the buttock, where a crease might be, to support the buttock. Brazilian buttocks age more gracefully because they are supported by fat below them and are thus less likely to droop. The ideal Brazilian butt is considerably larger than the present American ideal.

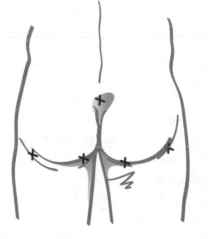

Typical needle incision sites for butt liposuction. Not all would be necessary in every case.

Before and after butt lipo-suction.

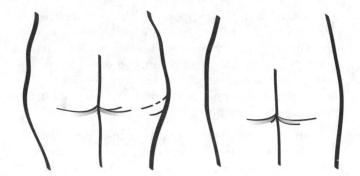

Some people think that liposuction will give their fanny a more desirable shape, but the procedure frequently leaves the fanny without adequate support and causes it to droop or sag even further than before. In these instances, fat transplantation is a more adequate remedy than liposuction.

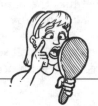

Wrinkle Ahead!

The idea of a buttock implant surfaces from time to time, but it is a procedure that is rarely done. The implant can be placed through a central incision between your buttocks, and if you didn't have to sit again, the procedure might have promise. Unfortunately, sitting seems to affect the implant badly over time because the pelvis doesn't provide a flat surface to place these implants on. Walking, bending, and sitting can result in movement of the implant. Gel implants can break in this area and are not used at all anymore. If a solid or soft-solid implant is placed, they migrate over time. Although you can find surgeons who still perform buttocks-implant surgery, we do not recommend this surgery.

When Your Fanny Is on the Line

Your first line of defense against a drooping fanny is exercise. For the exercise to be effective, you have to isolate the buttock muscles. The simplest way to do this is to use a stepper and to put your weight on your heels, not your toes, when you are on the machine (getting on your toes works other muscles).

If you want someone to exercise your butt muscles for you, it can be done to a degree. If you go to a place like the Madame & Monsieur chain of electrical exercise palaces, you can get your gluteus maximus muscles to contract and to get bigger and toned.

Whether you exercise your butt on a stair stepper or via electrical stimulation, you are increasing the size of the muscle and reducing the amount of fat. The exercises alone should help support your butt and help keep it from drooping, but if the exercises don't help enough, then you are still building a muscular frame for your surgeon to work on. The surgeon can then add and subtract fat from the local region to create a shape or reduce the overall size.

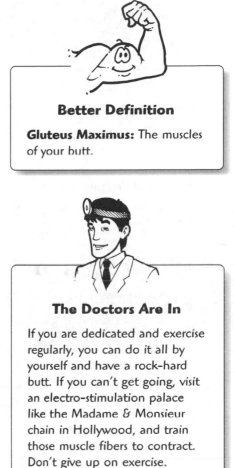

Better Definition

Gluteus Maximus: The muscles of your butt.

The Doctors Are In

If you are dedicated and exercise regularly, you can do it all by yourself and have a rock-hard butt. If you can't get going, visit an electro-stimulation palace like the Madame & Monsieur chain in Hollywood, and train those muscle fibers to contract. Don't give up on exercise.

Don't Expect Miracles Without Exercise and Diet

Liposuction combined with selective fat transplant (butt sculpting) is a fairly reliable procedure, but it must be followed by exercise and dietary restraint. If you are young and childless, you will have a better result than if you are older with more wear and tear from carrying children and weight fluctuation. If you don't intend to exercise, you will not do as well. Your exercise program should begin as you are planning surgery.

Buttock sculpting is not like a face-lift, where you can lie down and have fat, skin, and muscles lifted and trimmed as needed no matter what you weigh. Your surgeon will do all he or she can for you, but you will have to do your part by maintaining a healthy diet and exercise both before and after surgery.

Fanny Tucks Revisited

"Cut it off!" may be a valid wish, but the scars are horrendous and we don't recommend it. As a last resort, if you have very loose skin, the skin from your fanny can be trimmed. This is an old-fashioned fanny tuck. The scars will show in bathing suits and bedrooms.

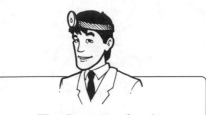

This operation is usually reserved for older people who have suffered from severe weight fluctuation. The surgery will leave large scars and the operation is irreversible. In other words, if you change your mind and you decide that you don't like the scars after your operation, there will be very little if anything that you or your surgeon will be able to do about it. Be sure that you can live with the outcome before you choose to move ahead with this operation or any other procedure that will improve the shape of your fanny.

There will be improvements surgically created for you, but this is clearly a bittersweet trade. You will be trading a less-than-ideal condition for a better condition, not an ideal one.

Telltale Signs of Candidacy

You are a candidate to surgically improve the shape of your fanny if ...

➤ Your fanny begins to lose its shape.

➤ Your fanny begins to sag or droop a little.

➤ Your fanny fat begins to empty from age and leave loose skin.

➤ Your fanny has excess skin from severe weight fluctuation.

➤ Your fanny hangs below the upper back crease of your leg.

➤ You are unable to distinctly define your fanny from the upper back part of your leg.

➤ You want a larger fanny.

➤ You want a smaller fanny.

➤ You want a rounder fanny.

➤ You want a tighter fanny.

➤ You want people to stop looking and laughing at your fanny.

If you can relate to any of the above prerequisites, you can probably benefit from having some cosmetic improvement made to your rear. Consider whether or not fat transplants, liposuction, or a full fanny-tuck operation would meet your cosmetic needs. Then consult with your cosmetic surgeon and ask for his or her opinion. You'll be glad you did.

The Cost of a New and Improved Fanny

Expect to pay between $5,00 and $6,000 for a fanny liposuction. Liposculpture, which includes fat transplants, will probably cost more.

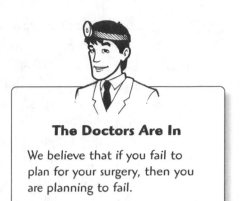

The Doctors Are In

We believe that if you fail to plan for your surgery, then you are planning to fail.

Cover Your Fanny!

After you have decided to go for one of these procedures, there are a few preoperative tips that you can consider in order to make your recovery period from fanny surgery run as smooth as possible. Remember, these tips will not only help you to feel better, they will also help you to heal better. Review the preoperative tips listed for you below and put them into practice before your surgery:

➤ Go on a high-protein, low-residue diet (low on fiber) or liquid diet so your bowel is cleaned out before buttock surgery.

➤ Use enemas. Enemas are sold over the counter at local drugstores and can help to cleanse you in preparation for your surgery.

➤ Don't have buttock surgery at the end of your menstrual cycle. You don't want any preoperative swelling in your body.

➤ Be sure to lose weight, not gain it, before surgery.

➤ Choose and maintain a realistic exercise program.

All of these tips will put your body in prime condition for your operation. Following these preoperative plans will help to make your surgery a success.

Fanny-Tuck Tips

This is not the longest recovery that there is from a surgery, but it certainly is the most delicate one! The postoperative period from any kind of fanny surgery is different than other types of recoveries because your fanny is a muscle group that you use every minute of the day. Whether you are sitting, standing, walking, or bending, you are using and can always feel your fanny. So, making yourself as comfortable as possible during your postoperative period is the number one goal. Here are some of our recommendations for an easy and uncomplicated recovery period:

➤ You need a lounge chair you can slouch in when you aren't in bed.

➤ Plan to walk. Bring a friend and something to sit on (you won't sit for long) if you become suddenly tired.

➤ You can shower, particularly if your wounds are sealed, with cyanoacrylate.

➤ Avoid bathing in the tub. The dirty water can infect your stitches.

➤ Take a week off work: Such a week begins on the Friday before the weekend, and includes the ending weekend as well. You will need the extra time.

➤ Don't plan on driving the first week. Have someone else drive and sit on pillows in the passenger seat. Recline the seat so you are in a lounging position. This will put more pressure on your back and less pressure on your fanny.

➤ Engage in nonstrenuous activities like reading, watching television, or surfing the Internet during the week to combat the boredom of being restricted to your home or care facility.

➤ Sleep as much as you can. Growth hormone, which helps you heal, is secreted when you sleep.

➤ Don't forget to eat regularly! You burn a lot of calories when you heal, so don't deprive yourself because you are too tired to eat.

➤ Stay out of the tanning booth for the first six months because the rays tend to prolong the bruising and also can delay skin contraction.

These are the most effective ways to ensure a safe and speedy recovery. We recommend that you follow all of these postoperative tips and follow up with your surgeon for a checkup to see how you are healing after a week or two. If you've had a full fanny tuck, your doctor will probably want to keep a close eye on your results. Plan to have someone drive you to one or two follow-up visits. You will want to be exceedingly careful to keep your incisions clean and avoid putting unnecessary pressure on your fanny. You can bet your backside that all of these tips will help you to recover quickly and without any unnecessary pain.

The Least You Need to Know

➤ Be weight stable or lose weight before surgery.

➤ Plan to maintain your surgical results through diet and exercise.

➤ Consider a full fanny tuck only as a last resort.

➤ If you're having fat transplanted, make sure that your doctor does not take fat from your stomach.

➤ Avoid driving for the first week of your recovery.

Part 5

Extremities and Other Things

Up to this point we've discussed several of the most popular surgeries that are available today. However, there are some operations that have been around for quite a while that are not as common but can still be just as effective in improving your appearance. There are also some surgeries past and present that promise to alter your appearance for the better but in actuality are unsafe, ineffective, and should be avoided. The chapters in this section will outline what options are available for thighs, arms, calves, and penises. Most importantly, they will tell you which operations are useful and which ones should be avoided at all costs!

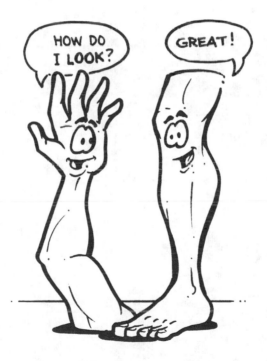

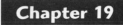

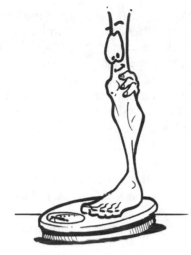

Chapter 19

Thinning Your Thighs

In This Chapter

➤ Why your thighs tend to accumulate fat

➤ What liposuction options are available for your legs and thighs

➤ Determining whether you're a good candidate for liposuction

➤ What you can expect to pay for thinner thighs

Big thighs are tough customers, no question about it. You can have the greatest-looking body, but if you've got flabby thighs, then it pretty much ruins you for swimsuit season. Fortunately, there are a number of remedies available to help you put your thighs into swimsuit-ready shape.

Although thighs are the most common problem areas of legs, we've also got solutions for fatty lower legs or ankles or knees. If you take the time and plan well, in just a few short months you will be looking your absolute best in clothes you would never have considered wearing before.

Look at My Eyes, not My Thighs

If you are one of those people who wish that others paid more attention to your eyes than the condition of your thighs, then you are probably right for this surgery. As a

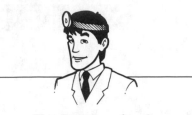

matter of fact, if you have legs that are in any kind of unsatisfactory shape to you—including unwanted fat in your thighs, knees, ankles, and even calves—you are a likely candidate for the treatments discussed in this chapter. Frequently, a well-structured leg is masked by fat deposits. Fat deposits can develop in all variations at the thighs, knees, and ankles.

Why Thighs?

Women's thighs naturally harbor both estrogen and proteins that contribute to unshapely legs. By reducing the mass at the thigh, you have less estrogen on board which makes your dieting and exercising more effective.

Pulling Your Leg ... for Real

There are more options available today for women who want to improve the look of their thighs and legs than ever before. If you've tried thinning your thighs through diet and exercise and haven't had any luck, then you might be a good candidate for upper-thigh liposuction or leg reshaping. These thigh-thinning surgeries are popular because women who already have firm, well-shaped legs and are thin can wear just about anything and look great after their operation! There is usually no need to camouflage any part of the leg except for the purpose of modesty, because the "trouble areas" have been instantly removed. Read on to find out about thigh liposuction and reshaping.

Leg Liposuction

Leg liposuction is a common procedure that produces dramatic results. We've described how liposuction works in general in Chapter 17, "Meeting in the Middle: Liposuction of the Midsection," and in this chapter we'll focus on liposuction of the legs.

Circumferential Liposuction

Circumferential liposuction is a fairly new technique that is a popular and a successful choice for thinning your thighs and legs. Small incision sites are made in strategic areas around your thighs in order to suction fat from all around your leg.

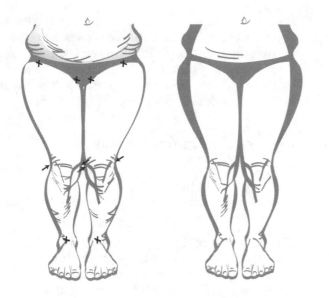

Before and after a full leg liposuction. Notice the incision marks at the upper legs (just under the bikini line), the knees, and the ankles.

If you only have portions of your legs liposuctioned, then you risk having a noticeable dent where the fat was removed. This is why we recommend that you have an entire area liposuctioned at one time. For example, if you have fatty legs beginning at the knee all the way up to the hip, you can have your doctor start liposuctioning from just below your knees, have him shape your knees and leg, and complete the surgery by having your upper leg and adjacent hip liposuctioned. Remember, there is a limit to how much fat you can have removed at one time: no more than nine pounds of fat.

A prolonged recovery may be necessary after a full-circumference liposuction in order for the fluid and swelling to be reduced.

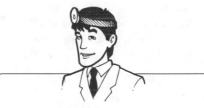

The Doctors Are In

As with all surgery that requires liposuction, you'll need to lose weight, be losing weight, or be weight stable prior to this surgery.

Spot Liposuction of the Legs—Leg Reshaping

People who have thin legs and thighs with only small deposits of fat are good candidates for what is called "spot liposuction." This procedure focuses only on particular spots of fat and is commonly performed at the thighs, knees, and ankles.

Most candidates for spot liposuction have a well-shaped lower leg that allows this surgery to stop at or below the knee, but if your calf is heavy (from fat depots), then fat above and below your calf can be sculpted along with your ankle.

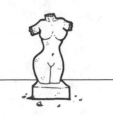

If your calf is thick due to muscle instead of fat, then liposuction will not be effective. Cosmetic surgeons are developing muscle-reduction procedures, but they are new and experimental and we don't recommend that anyone have such procedures. Don't be ashamed of those muscles—show them off with pride!

Liposuction Incisions

The most up-to-date approach to liposuction is with a puncture wound or very tiny incision, and most entry sites are well hidden in the groin, the buttock crease, and creases in the knee and ankle.

The results of leg liposuction can be dramatic! If any area of your leg is a candidate for liposuction, we recommend that you have it treated early and all at once. What are you waiting for? Swimsuit season is right around the corner!

Go Figure!

When most patients have a full-circumferential liposuction performed to reshape their legs, they tend to experience a continued generalized weight loss over the months following surgery. While this weight loss is possibly due to decreased estrogen (and fat-sparing proteins), the details of this phenomenon are not clearly understood by medical experts. But what experts do know is that you can anticipate losing weight after surgery!

Possible Side Effects

The success of liposuction depends on your skin's ability to contract. Skin has a tendency to contract by itself naturally. When your skin doesn't contract, it is usually because it has lost its elasticity from the aging process, sun damage, or from being overly stretched during pregnancy or chronic weight fluctuation.

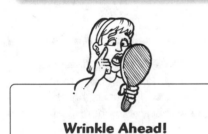

Wrinkle Ahead!

We don't recommend that you undergo any muscle-reduction procedures, which are new and experimental. If you have muscular legs, don't try to hide them; instead, take pride in them and show them off with impunity!

If your skin does not contract naturally, then it may drape or hang in an unusual-looking way after liposuction surgery. It can also develop an unnatural appearance if your remaining fat cells above the operated site hang downward and crease the structures below it. In these cases, a small additional liposuction can help to redrape your skin. The slight reduction in content under your skin may permit it to contract. Sometimes this will cause your skin to drape where you want it to drape. But remember, your age and your general skin condition are factors in whether or not your skin will contract.

Getting a Leg up on Leg Liposuction

If you're considering a thigh lift or leg lift, keep in mind that you need to be fit and cannot be clinically obese (overweight by 20 percent of the average for a person who is your same age and height).

One of the many ironies about fat and weight loss is that the presence of thigh fat actually makes it harder for people who diet to lose weight. If you have fat thighs, we recommend that you reduce your caloric intake and *increase* exercise, which will help you increase your muscle mass and increase your resting metabolism rate. A speedier metabolism should help you lose weight and thus prepare you for liposuction surgery.

Your doctor will also want to check your hormone levels and circulating protein levels to make sure they are at a surgery-friendly level, otherwise complications could arise. Your doctor will let you know what these levels should be, as they vary depending on your biological makeup.

Here are some other things you should know in order to determine if you are a good candidate for leg liposuction surgery:

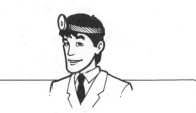

The Doctors Are In

We suggest that you don't put your liposuction off too long, or your skin might not contract enough or drape well.

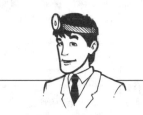

The Doctors Are In

Proper nutrition and maintaining a healthy and active lifestyle require a permanent shift in the way you view food and exercise. You may need the help of professionals in order to achieve your goals.

➤ You need to receive a clean bill of health from your physician. That means you must be diabetes-free, your hypertension must be under control, and all major psychological issues (anorexia, bulimia, body dysmorphia, etc.) need to be ruled out as motivating factors for this operation. You need to be of sound mind, free from major depression and anxiety, and not be impulsively looking for a quick "pick me up" that you might regret after your operation is over.

➤ Any plans for pregnancy need to be postponed until you have made a complete recovery. You don't want to jeopardize your baby or cause other health risks.

➤ Any kind of surgery that involves liposuction, especially leg surgery, is going to require you to lose weight as you prepare for surgery. Intervention with pharmaceutical weight-loss drugs seems to lead to rebound weight gain. We suggest you rely on other methods of losing weight, like counseling to help you change the way you view food and exercise, consulting with a dietician to help you come up

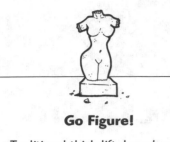

Go Figure!

Traditional thigh lifts have been completely abandoned except for people who have had severe weight fluctuation and want to have the excess skin removed after they have gotten down to their goal weight.

with a meal plan that would be realistic for you to follow, and joining a gym to get a regular dose of cardiovascular exercise like walking, swimming, or biking.

What's a Thinner Thigh Worth To You?

Thinner thighs, via liposuction, will generally cost between $6,000 and $8,000.

Now That You've Decided To Have Liposuction ...

Once you've determined that you are ready to have leg liposuction, you need to make an appointment with your cosmetic surgeon to discuss the procedure and then take some time to prepare for the surgery. Here are some things your doctor will likely want you to do before you come in for your procedure:

➤ You'll need to have blood taken ahead of surgery so it is available in case it is needed during your surgery, which is common with liposuction procedures. You can collect as much as two to three units of whole blood in two-week intervals. You'll need to wait two weeks after the last donation before having surgery in order to build your blood supply back up. Whole blood can be stored in refrigeration for the first 30 days and will need to be frozen after that.

➤ You already need to be on an exercise program that you can realistically begin and maintain starting a month after your surgery. This is a standard part of an active and healthy lifestyle. Join your local gym or talk with a trainer about developing a realistic workout program.

➤ You'll need to be well rested pre- and postoperatively. Avoid overscheduling yourself before and after your surgery. We suggest that you schedule a three-week recovery period. Make necessary arrangements ahead of time. Many people go back to work in 10 to 14 days with a leotard or tight-fitting bodysuit under their clothes to reinforce a speedy contraction of their skin.

➤ You need to arrange to have someone with you all or most of the time for the first week of your recovery because you will be sore and unable to do anything for anybody, including yourself. You will need help with dressing, sitting, standing, lying down, getting up, and bending down!

➤ Plan not to eat food that is preserved because it can slow down your healing process by causing swelling. Look through your cupboards and refrigerator and put these foods in a designated area with a reminder note to yourself not to eat them after surgery. Otherwise, you may be so groggy after your surgery that you will forget to avoid these foods.

Take these tips to heart and your recovery period will be as smooth and easy as possible.

Break a Leg!

Once you've had your surgery performed, plan to rest for at least two weeks, but preferably three. You'll definitely want to wait until you are relatively pain-free to return to your daily activities. Also, consider these postoperative tips for a smooth recovery period:

➤ Set your house up so you know where your antibiotics, pain medications, and protein powder are located. You won't be hungry for a few days, but high-protein intake is very important. You need to have protein powder ready for this.

➤ Be ready to eat a salt-restricted diet. This isn't a time to diet, but it is also not a time to eat salty foods like bacon or pizza, either. Salt will cause you to swell and will affect how well you heal.

➤ Your legs will be stiff, and you'll need someone to assist you in walking to the bathroom.

➤ Do not get into a tub that you won't be able to get out of by yourself. We recommend that you shower instead of bathe so that your incisions do not get infected by dirty bathtub water. If you shower after the first few days, be sure to have a stable stool to sit on.

➤ Sudden fatigue is common. You'll need constant supervision and to sit down frequently. If you don't walk and move around, you can develop circulatory issues and clots. This is true of any surgery. Sit in a chair for meals and snacks.

➤ Don't tire yourself out with guests. Rent some of your favorite videos to watch. Stay quiet, be still, and rest!

These are all the facts you need to know from the beginning to the end of your thigh-thinning surgery. Break a leg!

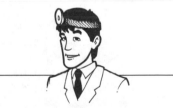

The Doctors Are In

Unshapely legs, thighs, knees, and ankles all have remedies available today that were never dreamed of before. You can pretty much fix what you need to without the scars seen in earlier days.

The Least You Need to Know

➤ Make sure you don't have a psychological disorder such as anorexia or bulemia.

➤ Don't sign up for a little and expect a lot—if you want your whole leg to look trimmer, then have your whole leg liposuctioned.

➤ Get a clean bill of health before surgery.

➤ Be weight stable or losing weight when you have your procedure. Do not go in gaining weight under the assumption that it will all get suctioned out.

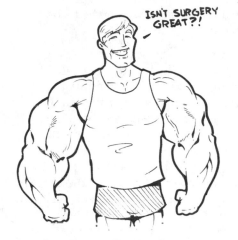

ISN'T SURGERY GREAT?!

Chapter 20

To Arms! To Arms! Arm Reshaping

In This Chapter

➤ What you can do for your flabby arms

➤ Deciding between spot- and full-circumference liposuction

➤ When should you start stopping the flab

➤ When liposuction isn't enough

Chubby arms might be cute on babies, but once you're an adult, they're not so cute anymore. As a matter of fact, flabby arms can be downright embarrassing if you want to wear sleeveless or short-sleeve tops. For those of you who want to cosmetically re-shape your arms, this chapter is for you!

The Right to Bare Arms

We've identified two types of people who can benefit from arm-sculpting surgery if they want to bare their arms in sleeveless tops and look their absolute best:

1. Women who have baby-fat depots in their arms that didn't recede or even increased at puberty.

2. Women who have experienced extreme weight fluctuation and can't lose the excess fat in their arms even after they've lost other weight.

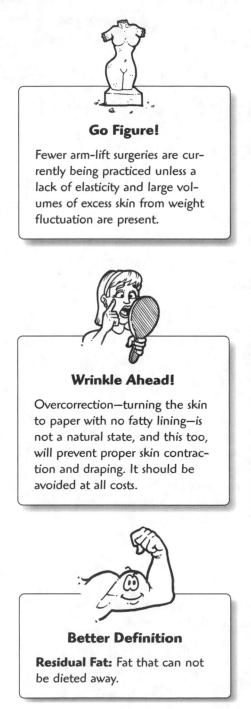

Go Figure!

Fewer arm-lift surgeries are currently being practiced unless a lack of elasticity and large volumes of excess skin from weight fluctuation are present.

Wrinkle Ahead!

Overcorrection—turning the skin to paper with no fatty lining—is not a natural state, and this too, will prevent proper skin contraction and draping. It should be avoided at all costs.

Better Definition

Residual Fat: Fat that can not be dieted away.

If your arms match either of these types of descriptions, then you are a good candidate for the techniques discussed in this chapter.

If you are like most women who seek out this surgery, you want to know exactly where the fat is located that can be removed from your arm. Fatty deposits tend to develop and collect at the upper part of the arm between the lower shoulder and the elbow for many women. Although this area is usually the space that women discuss with their surgeons when they talk about arm-reshaping surgery, the area around the elbow and sometimes the lower arms (below the elbow) can be addressed in extreme cases. Shoulders can also be treated. You can have all areas cosmetically improved since fat deposits or loose skin can develop in all parts of your arms depending on your development, age, and weight history.

You'll increase your chances of having a successful surgery by having the operation performed when you are younger, because younger skin tends to contract better than older skin. It has a certain "snap" to it!

Liposuction Options

Since the 1980s, liposuction of the arm has widely replaced arm-lifting surgery, because liposuction can remove substantial volumes of fat through very small and sometimes unnoticeable incisions and allow the skin to contract naturally. It avoids the long incisions that resulted from old arm lifts and allows you to heal much more quickly. (See Chapter 17, "Meeting in the Middle: Liposuction of the Midsection" for a detailed description of liposuction.)

It is *residual fat* at the arms that is usually responsible for dragging the skin downward or that causes youthful skin to drape in an unfavorable way. This is why more and more women are finding that liposuction, even if it has to be done in stages, is a more desirable treatment for arm resculpting than arm lifts. In fact, liposuction of the arms is the new treatment of choice for arm resculpting today.

Spot Liposuction

If fat deposits did not develop in your arms during puberty and it was a development that occurred in early or later adulthood, you might be an excellent candidate for minor liposuction surgery, sometimes called "spot liposuction." Minor liposuction can be performed in stages to tease older skin into contracting gradually and resculpt the shape of your arms. This way, a large demand for contraction is not placed on skin that only has a minimal ability to contract. Contraction can be achieved in realistic and easy-to-manage doses by having small amounts of liposuction performed over a course of several sessions.

When to Bare Arms?

Many women think that they should wait until their arms are so out of shape that they just can't stand it anymore. Not true! If you wait, you might perpetuate your condition, because early treatment can prevent increased fat from forming. Also, the longer you wait to get the procedure done, the more chance you face of losing elasticity in your skin.

We recommend that you have this surgery performed early if you are in fact a candidate. It will prevent your condition from accelerating and your skin will contract better after your surgery. It can also help you to become a candidate for just a minor touch-up liposuction instead of a full arm-lift operation later on.

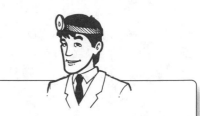

The Doctors Are In

Liposuction is not the first line of defense for generalized obesity. Obesity is a biochemical problem that should be corrected or controlled through counseling, medication, diet, and/or exercise. Liposuction should only be used as an additional treatment to improve your appearance and quality of life.

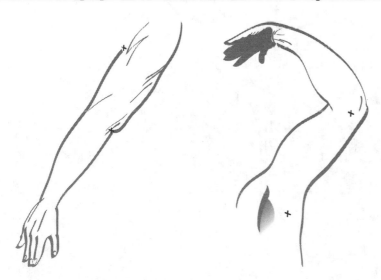

Typical arms suitable for liposuction, showing incision sites.

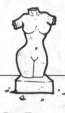

Go Figure!

Skin that has an ability to contract easily usually looks full, smooth, and firm. Skin that does not contract easily usually looks less full, less smooth, and less firm.

When the skin around the arm does not contract easily, the surrounding skin on other parts of the body usually suffers from the same poor elasticity. This means that you can still have arm-resculpting surgery on your arms even if your skin does not easily contract. The results of your surgery will still look natural and won't be out of keeping with the rest of your body. After all, any improvement that is made is still an improvement at any age. And would you really want to have 20-year-old arms on a body that still looks 40 or 50?

This is the definition you can expect after your arm liposuction. Some people are surprised when they can see their muscles.

A Few Words About Old-Fashioned Arm Lifts

The 1970s were an exuberant time in the field of cosmetic surgery. Body-lifting techniques were proposed and attempted in operating rooms across the country. Arm lifts quickly became an available and moderately popular surgery. They were commonly performed in conjunction with thigh, leg, and/or torso lifts on out-of-shape patients who needed them.

Ugly Incisions

There is no place to adequately place incisions during an arm-lift operation so that they will not be visible later on. Because of the scarring, arm lifts should only be used as a last resort to improve someone's appearance after obesity has appropriately been treated with diet, exercise, counseling, and appropriate medication (if necessary).

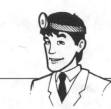

The Doctors Are In

We consider arm lifts to be a last resort for arm shaping. We recommend more preventative or corrective methods such as diet or exercise and having this surgery only when all other methods have failed. (The only exception to this rule is congenital fat pads that develop at puberty that don't respond to this). We predict that less and less of these procedures will be done, as more and more generations are well informed, practice nutritious eating, and maintain healthy and active lifestyles.

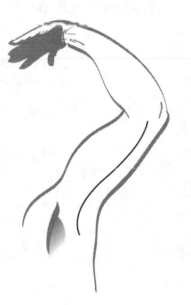

This is the kind of scarring that results from a traditional arm lift. There is no good way to hide the scar, and arm lifts should only be considered as a last resort if the skin will not contract after weight loss.

It's Probably Not Worth It

We recommend that you weigh old-fashioned arm-lifting surgery (not liposuction) very carefully. Many women say "I just want to look better in clothes" and they report that they don't care about the scars that this surgery will inevitably cause. When they say this, they think about wearing sheer tops with no sleeves. They soon find the scars that this surgery leaves are much more visible than what they initially anticipated. This can precipitate a series of events: They have their scars revised. They have their scars tattooed in attempts to conceal them. They become experts in waterproof makeup.

We don't recommend arm lifts (except as a last resort for those who have completely lost skin elasticity from age or severe weight fluctuation) for a variety of reasons. The main reason is that the scars are obviously visible. A true arm lift treats the skin but not the fat, and recurrence of fat can be possible both at the surgery site and adjacent to it. This almost always requires more surgery and creates even more scars. In plain words, it is not enough cure for the scar you receive. The price is just too high!

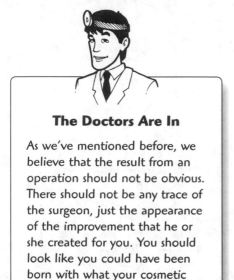

The Doctors Are In

As we've mentioned before, we believe that the result from an operation should not be obvious. There should not be any trace of the surgeon, just the appearance of the improvement that he or she created for you. You should look like you could have been born with what your cosmetic surgeon gave you.

How to Get Better Results Without Ugly Scars

Another reason we usually do not recommend an arm-lift operation is that the need for it can be prevented or treated through diet and exercise. We suggest this operation be reserved for those who have successfully treated obesity and need cosmetic improvement, not as a measure for treating obesity. If you have fatty deposits in your arms, we recommend that you practice preventative methods (like diet and exercise) and then have a less obvious and less invasive liposuction surgery performed to cosmetically improve the appearance of your arms.

Arm lifts are not a first line of defense and should be considered a last resort with many drawbacks that must be clearly understood. There is nothing that can reverse the problems associated with arm lifts.

How Much for New Arms?

The total cost for arm liposuction is $5,000–$6,000. A traditional arm lift generally costs about the same.

Get Ready!

Get ready for some preoperative tips you'll need to keep in mind before moving ahead with arm liposuction.

This can be a painful surgery if you don't follow our suggestions. Make your operation and recovery period an agreeable one, and take the following advice to heart:

Don't fill yourself up with "feel goods" and anticoagulants before surgery.

Be sure the doctor knows what medications you are taking and confirms that they do not conflict with the anesthesia or surgery to be performed. Ask your surgeon when your usual medications can be resumed.

Know your allergy history.

Tell your doctor everything that you are allergic to, sensitive to, or have an unnatural reaction to (for instance, some people have unusual responses like becoming more alert after drinking a beverage that contains caffeine) even if you think it is unimportant. It could save your life!

Schedule someone to supervise you after your surgery.

This may be a spouse, friend, older child, or other loved one. This person's goal should be to help you to limit your movement to necessary tasks that only you can perform (like getting up to go to the restroom or showering) and to help you reserve your range of motion (have him or her hand you things instead of reaching for them yourself).

Don't go into arm-liposuction surgery dehydrated.

You must avoid eating or drinking 24 hours before surgery, but the days and weeks prior should not be spent on a crash diet that is going to dehydrate you. Dehydration can lead to sudden fatigue after surgery. Surgery often compromises your stamina because healing puts an extra demand for energy on your body. You should be losing weight, but not in drastic fashion the night before surgery.

Plan to have general anesthesia during your liposuction surgery.

Incisions that will be well hidden after your surgery will be stretched during the procedure to adequately suction all of the fat. Local anesthesia may not provide enough pain relief, and you will not want to be conscious to see all positions your arms will be placed in during your operation so that your surgeon can appropriately treat the area.

Know what an arm looks like postoperatively before your surgery.

Ask your doctor to see some postoperative pictures. This way, you can anticipate what you will look like and will be assured that your results are normal for someone who has just had surgery. Not everyone knows what a normal arm looks like when the fat is suctioned. It can be quite startling.

During your preoperative consultation, you might want to plan to have some of your fat that is suctioned from your surgery transplanted to another area of your body.

You can have it injected into your lips or laugh lines. After all, waste not, want not. Put your fat to good use—in the places where you want it to be! You can have this done at the same time as your operation.

Be weight stable.

Come in for surgery being weight stable, ideally at a lower end of your tolerable weight range.

If you have recently lost weight, allow plenty of time for your skin to contract before scheduling surgery.

This will spare the length of incision used in liposuction or arm lifting, if you have to resort to the latter. Some people respond well to sequential reduction liposuction of the arm, and everyone who is overweight can benefit from a preoperative diet!

These simple and easy suggestions can help you to be in the best shape for your arm-reshaping surgery.

After the Party's Over

OK, so the party's over. You've had your operation. Now the recovery begins! This is usually a painful recovery period because you use your arms almost as much as you use your legs during an average day. Obviously, you'll want to use your arms as little as possible after your surgery. Here are a few postoperative tips to help you maximize your arm-lift results and minimize the use of your arms after your surgery.

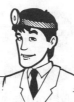

The Doctors Are In

If you watch your diet by limiting sugar and fats and ingesting high levels of protein, lots of antioxidants, and vitamins for your skin with cell stimulator, collagen stimulator, and phyto-estrogen, you can maintain the firmness and appearance of your upper arm and delay the outward signs of aging. Some people who are diligent and patient can reverse some of the appearances of aging. Wearing sunscreen and avoiding tanning beds can also help the condition and appearance of your skin. Remember, all results of cosmetic surgery depend on the resilience of your skin and its ability to heal.

Plan for comfort!

Have the person supervising you cook your meals so you won't have to cook or grocery shop when you get hungry. Let this other person do whatever you usually do for yourself or others until you feel better (usually a couple of days). There are no medals for bravery. If you don't rest and challenge your healing time, it can take longer, which is just the opposite of what you want to accomplish.

Wear a long sleeve leotard top.

It should be firm on your arms and fit your torso well. You can't get sleeves on regular clothes to stay in place, and wrapping your arms with bandages will be uneven and contribute marks to the healing process. Be sure that your leotard has long sleeves. Otherwise the short sleeves or three-quarter sleeves will cause marks or uneven healing.

Eat a high-protein, low-salt diet.

You need energy and protein as building blocks to heal. The early contraction of skin is both desirable and comfortable. If you eat a lot of foods with salt, you tend to retain fluid and swell. This swelling will be the greatest at the fresh surgery site. Swelling in this area delays the contraction of the skin.

Don't ice your arms.

Ice doesn't help that much after this kind of surgery, and it may annoy you. When you have surgery, salt is retained the first two days or so and creates swelling. Icing the arms constricts the capillaries, slowing protein loss into the operated area, and can prevent your swelling from decreasing.

Use magnets to reduce bruising.

Tesla (who worked with Thomas Edison) described a magnetic field that does promote the healing process; when tested in the lab, this field helps cells divide. When a magnet is placed on surgical wounds, negative side against the skin and positive side up, the bruising fades faster than adjacent untreated areas. Some surgeons have magnetic fields available, and if you need them, they can also be purchased from alternative medicine sources or medical supply sources. We are not advocating using magnets indefinitely, but in the first week or two it certainly helps with the three things on your mind: healing, swelling, and pain.

Elevate your arms above heart level and do not sleep on them.

This will keep the natural swelling down.

Stay out of the sun or tanning booth.

The sun's rays slow skin contraction and can make bruises last longer. The tanning booth uses UVA rays. It is the UVB that burns. The UVA is associated with skin cancer. UVA and UVB both make bruising "set" (take to the area like a dye), sometimes permanently, after this or any surgery. The sun and tanning booths delay the process of smoothing and bruising and delays the swelling going down. This seems to delay healing.

These suggestions are everything you need to know for a successful recovery period. Follow these tips and you can't go wrong. As a matter of fact, you'll be waving your arms with delight in no time. Well, almost no time!

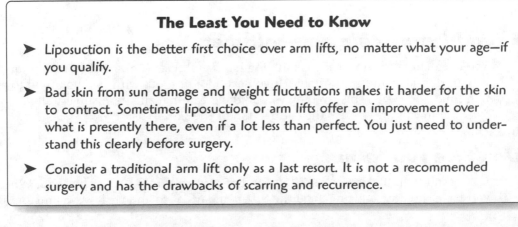

The Least You Need to Know

➤ Liposuction is the better first choice over arm lifts, no matter what your age—if you qualify.

➤ Bad skin from sun damage and weight fluctuations makes it harder for the skin to contract. Sometimes liposuction or arm lifts offer an improvement over what is presently there, even if a lot less than perfect. You just need to understand this clearly before surgery.

➤ Consider a traditional arm lift only as a last resort. It is not a recommended surgery and has the drawbacks of scarring and recurrence.

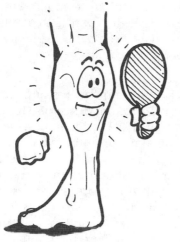

Chapter 21

A New Leg to Stand On: Calf Implants

In This Chapter

➤ Taking a look at calf-implantation techniques

➤ How to prepare for surgery

➤ What to expect after your surgery

Calf implants? It's true, some people desire more shapely calves and are willing to undergo a reconstructive surgery and implants in order to get the look they desire.

We won't pull your leg about calf-implantation surgery—it's painful! Actually, it's one of the more painful cosmetic procedures, and even with an adequate supply of the strongest pain relievers, the recovery period can be excruciating. You must really want shapelier calves in order for the recovery period to be worth the discomfort you will experience. This is not a procedure for a novice or anyone who thinks that he or she will have surgery one day and be back to work or the gym the next day, or even the next week.

Having a Leg To Stand On

If you want to have a great set of legs to stand on, you'll need to know which surgical technique is the best one for you when you decide to have calf-implant surgery performed.

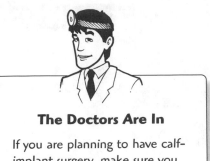

Although many doctors use various techniques for calf-implantation surgery, the best way is a combination of techniques that have been perfected by Dr. Adrian Aiache of Beverly Hills, Calif.

Dr. Aiache is recognized by some in the field of cosmetic surgery for developing two new instruments, the ball dissector and the hammer dissector. These instruments help to prevent the occasional muscular laceration and the occasional uncontrollable bleeding that were problematic with other instruments used by surgeons during calf-implantation surgery in the past. Dr. Aiache is also credited with creating six sizes of semisolid silicone implants that allow patients to choose the size of implant that would best fit their body type and give them a fuller, more natural appearance. Because the implants are semisolid, they are pliable enough to be cut with a scalpel so that they can be reduced and fitted perfectly to each person's individual need.

Currently, surgeons all over the world use different versions of these semisolid silicone implants to create custom-made calves for their patients. It's important to keep in mind that only semisolid silicone implants are used in the United States today. If your doctor uses anything else, that doctor is not for you!

Your calves have two muscles on either side. So, in order to achieve a more natural-looking appearance, Dr. Aiache's surgical technique uses two semisolid silicone implants to accentuate these two muscles and give the appearance of fuller and shapelier calves. Once your implants have been satisfactorily chosen and taped to the outside of your legs to give you an idea of where your implants will go and how your legs will look after your procedure, your surgery will begin.

The Procedure

The calf-implant procedure can be performed with either local or general anesthesia. Once you've been properly anesthetized, your surgeon will use a marker to make a horizontal outline along the crease of the back of your knees to designate where the incisions for the insertion of your implants will be located. Then, your surgeon will outline where the implants will be placed in your calves. Two pockets will be created inside your calves in order to make room for your new implants.

After the incision has been made, your surgeon will use an instrument to separate muscle from tissue in your calves to create the necessary pockets into which your implants will be inserted. Your new implants will be inserted through the small incisions in the back of your knees and massaged into place on both sides of your calves. Your incision then will be properly sutured. You need to stay in recovery a minimum of two hours however, some people require a longer stay. Usually, no hospitalization is necessary!

This procedure is relatively quick and easy. Best of all, you'll end up with great-looking calves, and if size is important to you, you can still continue to build up your calf muscles even after your surgery!

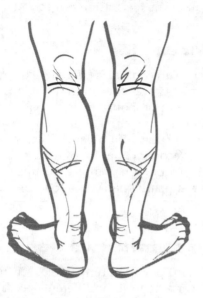

The incision sites for calf implants.

The location of calf implants.

The Cost of More Shapely or Muscular Legs

Calf surgery isn't cheap, but it's worth it for some people. The estimated cost of surgery, including anesthesia and operating room expenses, is $10,000.

Getting a Leg up on Surgery

Before you decide that calf-implantation surgery is right for you, you'll need to get a leg up on the surgery by finding out all of the facts. Here's what you'll need to know.

Listen to your doctor's advice.

When most people walk into a cosmetic surgeon's office for any kind of implant surgery, they usually want the biggest implants available, even if they would look ridiculously out of proportion with the rest of their body. The same is true with calf implants. When you choose the size of your calf implants, listen carefully to your doctor's recommendation of what size and shape would look best on your calves, especially if they are smaller implants than what you originally had in mind.

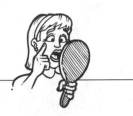

Wrinkle Ahead!

Cosmetic surgeons who have performed numerous calf-implantation surgeries know that the larger the implant is, the larger the risk is for complications. If an implant is too large for your body, you could run the serious risk of injuring the nerves in your calves that could cause temporary or permanent nerve damage. Too large of an implant could also result in infection, an impaired ability to walk, and a host of other adverse side effects. Listen to your doctor's advice when selecting the size of your implants and choose wisely!

Plan to take two weeks off work.

You'll need plenty of time to recover from this surgery. Everyone heals at different speeds, but most people are able to go back to work and return to most of their daily activities after 10 to 14 days. In case you heal a little slower than the average person, plan to take two weeks of recovery time off from work.

Make sure help is available.

Unlike most cosmetic procedures, calf-implantation surgery temporarily restricts your mobility. It will be difficult to walk during the first week of your recovery and you will need assistance to do simple tasks like getting in and out of bed, taking a shower, getting dressed, etc. Be sure to plan ahead and schedule a trusted friend or family member to be with you for at least the first week after your surgery.

Stop all steroid use.

Stop all use of medications that might complicate surgery. Some medications, including steroids, can cause bleeding during or after surgery. This can complicate your surgery and slow down your recovery process. Other medications can have other adverse effects during and after your surgery, too.

Make sure that your medical doctor and your cosmetic surgeon are aware of all medications that you are taking, and ask if you should stop taking them prior to your surgery. Stop your medications only when your doctor has given his approval, and schedule your surgery far enough in advance so that your body will be free of any medications that would be counterproductive to your surgery and your recovery.

Avoid working out prior to surgery.

In order to get the best results, your calves should be in optimum condition for surgery. They should be relaxed and free of as much tension as possible. Intense workouts which focus on building up the calf muscles prior to your surgery would be counterproductive to your goal of relaxing the muscles and put you at risk for injuring your calves. For this reason, it is best that you stop working out your calf muscles two months prior to your procedure.

Avoid strenuous leg activity prior to surgery.

Be sure that your daily and recreational activities do not include any kind of exercises that require strenuous leg activities, such as running, hiking, or skiing. Activities that involve strenuous leg activity will not condition your legs for calf surgery and can put you at risk for injury. Be sure to avoid or restrict any kind of strenuous leg activity two months prior to surgery. In case you do become injured, two months should be adequate time for your legs to heal and be ready for your procedure.

For those who enjoy exercising and don't want to give up working out their calf muscles prior to surgery, there is good news! You can still practice stretching exercises up to the day of your surgery. So, if you love to exercise and you think it might

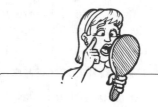

Wrinkle Ahead!

Avoid using steroids that are not prescribed by your doctor. Use or misuse of steroids can cause sever liver damage and a host of other adverse side-effects.

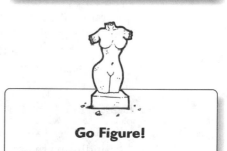

Go Figure!

Tense calf muscles or muscles that are injured do not leave your calves in the optimum condition for surgery.

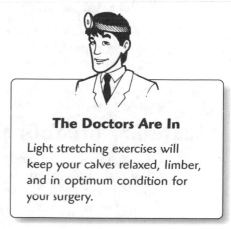

The Doctors Are In

Light stretching exercises will keep your calves relaxed, limber, and in optimum condition for your surgery.

help you to relax before your procedure, feel free to include some light stretching exercises in your daily activities up until your surgery date.

Wear comfortable clothes.

Wear clothes that are as comfortable as you would like to feel before, during, and after your surgery. Wearing clothes that are easy to put on and take off will make getting ready to go to and from your cosmetic surgeon's office a quicker trip. Be sure the clothes that you select are casual and have a relaxed fit (like elastic skirts or jogging pants with an elastic waistband) so that you can move around easily.

Stop tanning one month before surgery.

When you tan, you run the risk of getting a sunburn. Sunburned skin or skin that is peeling is more difficult to operate on and can cause increased discomfort during your recovery. In addition, it can cause the complexion of your skin to heal unevenly. For the sake of an easier surgery and a more comfortable recovery, avoid tanning for one month prior to your procedure.

Shave behind your knees two days before surgery

Freshly shaven legs can sometimes be raw, sensitive, and easily irritated. These can be difficult conditions to operate under. In order to optimize the condition of your skin for surgery, be sure to shave behind your knees (where the incisions will be made) two days prior to your surgery. Two days should also give your legs enough time to heal in case you suffer any small nicks or cuts from shaving.

Don't wax your legs right before surgery.

Waxing can frequently cause red, swollen, and bumpy skin. For optimum surgical conditions, your skin should be clean, clear, and smooth. Keep this in mind, and avoid waxing your legs right before surgery.

Remember all these facts, and everything will be just fine!

Standing on Your Own Two Feet

As we indicated at the outset of this chapter, calf-implantation surgery can be quite painful and full recovery can take quite some time. Read on and discover exactly what to anticipate during your recovery period from this operation before you decide it's right for you.

It will be difficult to walk for 7 to 10 days after surgery.

Incisions have been made in the back of your legs and muscles, and tissues in your calves have been separated in order to make room for your new implants. It will be completely natural and normal for you to experience moderate levels of discomfort immediately after your procedure.

You can anticipate having a difficult time walking for seven to ten days after your surgery. As the muscles and tissues adjust to your new implants and your body begins to heal, it will become easier for you to walk. Also, plan on staying in bed for the first 24 hours of your recovery so that your implants will not shift immediately after your surgery.

Walk with knees slightly bent.

By walking on your toes with your knees slightly bent, you can take the pressure off of your calf muscles. This will help to reduce any pain that you may be having and relieve your calves of any unnecessary strain. As you begin to feel more comfortable being on your feet, you can begin to bend your knees less and allow your calves to withstand the normal weight of your body when you walk.

Plan to walk in heeled shoes.

When you do begin to walk, wearing heeled shoes (pumps for women and dress shoes that slip on for men) will also help to take the pressure off your calf muscles. This will help to take the pressure off your calf muscles when you walk and redistribute the pressure of your body weight to the balls of your feet.

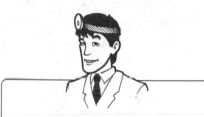

The Doctors Are In

If you have shoes with varying heel sizes (high, moderate, and low), you might want to start out wearing your shoes that have a higher heel on them and gradually work your way down to wearing shoes with a lower heel, until you can walk flat-footed without shoes.

Elevate your ankles.

While you are recovering from your surgery, you might be tempted to put your feet up and relax. Don't! Elevating your feet will cause the blood to rush to your calves and can cause increased swelling, soreness, and other complications. Instead, lie flat on your back and place a small pillow or rolled towel under your ankles (only) so that your calves are comfortably supported and your feet are not suspended higher than knee level. This will take the weight of your legs off of your calves and allow for an even and steady blood flow through out the lower parts of your body.

Bandages and ice are your friends.

Immediately following surgery, your legs will be wrapped from ankle to knee in an ACE bandage. This will help to reduce swelling and support the placement of your new implants. Stockings or socks may also be worn over the bandages to keep the bandages in place. In addition, you will want to ice your legs with bags of crushed ice or frozen peas to reduce inflammation.

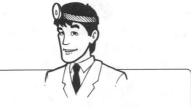

The Doctors Are In

Remember, bandages and ice are your friends! They will help to reduce swelling and inflammation from your surgery and aid in your recovery process. Plan to use bandages and ice for seven to ten days after your surgery (or as needed).

No bathing for one week.

Your stitches will be properly bandaged with surgical tape to protect them from infection. You may take the surgical tape off before you shower (if your doctor approves). You can shower after the first 24 hours of your surgery, if you have someone to help you. But you will want to avoid taking a bath until your stitches have properly healed, because sitting in dirty bathtub water will most likely infect your stitches. It will take approximately one week for your stitches to sufficiently heal.

So, wait seven days after your surgery before taking a bath and take showers instead during the first week of your recovery. Be sure to reapply your bandages after you've showered.

Use crutches for the first few days after surgery.

The first 24 hours of your recovery should be devoted to resting. After that, your goal is to learn to walk flat-footed again with as little pain as possible. Crutches will help.

Use crutches during the first few days of your recovery until you are able to walk without them. Your doctor will most likely have a pair that you can use. Use your crutches to let your calves gradually get used to supporting all of your body weight again. Remember, your goal is to walk flat-footed again with as little pain as possible (without the crutches).

Expect swollen and bruised calves for two to three weeks.

Keep in mind that some swelling and bruising is a natural response to surgery. The majority of the average person's swelling and bruising dissipates two to three weeks after surgery. Everyone heals at different speeds, so your swelling and bruising may dissipate a little slower or faster than the average person. Many people experience a continued decrease in swelling even months after their procedure.

Expect sore and stiff calves for three to four weeks after surgery.

As your body adjusts to its new implants, you may experience mild soreness and stiffness up to three to four weeks after your surgery. It will take awhile for your implants to feel like a natural part of your body. Expect your calves to be somewhat sore and stiff until the muscles and tissues in your legs adapt to your new implants. Like lip implants, calf implants can be felt and seen in very thin people.

Don't work out your calves for one to two months after surgery.

Once you're walking flat-footed again, you may feel like you're ready to get back to the gym. If you anticipate getting back to a regular workout schedule as soon as possible, wait four to eight weeks after your surgery before resuming any kind of weight training with your calves. Allow your calves enough time to get use to supporting the full weight of your body with the implants before adding extra weight or putting additional strain on your calves.

Avoid running for two to three months after surgery.

After eight to twelve weeks, your calves have probably had sufficient time to heal and get used to their new implants. They are ready to support additional weight and withstand strenuous movement like light jogging or running. With your doctor's approval, you can resume running eight to twelve weeks after surgery. Resuming any kind of running any earlier without your doctor's approval can place you at high risk for complications and impaired recovery.

Be sure to wait the recommended amount of time and to get your doctor's approval before you get out your jogging shoes!

In case of infection, call your doctor.

The four common signs of infection are pain, swelling, tenderness, and redness. Of course, you will probably experience some mild forms of some

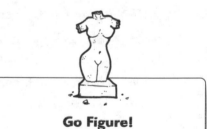

Go Figure!

With the recent developments in the field of cloning which makes replication of human tissue and organs possible, it makes sense to anticipate that it won't be long before you can have your own muscles reproduced and then implanted into your own body. If you are considering calf-implantation surgery, would you rather have semisolid silicone prostheses or your very own muscles inserted into your body? Which sounds better to you?

of these symptoms as a result of your surgery; it does not mean you have an infection, it just means you are experiencing some common reactions to surgery. Mild forms of these symptoms are natural. But if you are experiencing severe levels of pain, swelling, tenderness, and redness, to the point of unbearable pain or discomfort, you may very well have an infection. If you experience any of these symptoms to a degree that feels uncomfortable for you or seems unusual, call your doctor immediately.

These are all the things you can anticipate from calf-implantation surgery. All of these elements are important to anticipate and plan for if you decide to move ahead with calf-implantation surgery.

Calf implants aren't for everyone, but for people who desire more shapely or muscular-looking calves, they are one alternative.

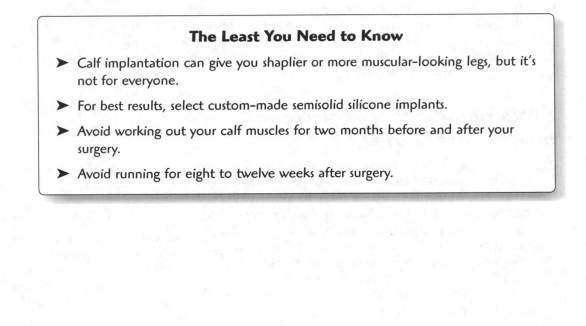

The Least You Need to Know

➤ Calf implantation can give you shaplier or more muscular-looking legs, but it's not for everyone.

➤ For best results, select custom-made semisolid silicone implants.

➤ Avoid working out your calf muscles for two months before and after your surgery.

➤ Avoid running for eight to twelve weeks after surgery.

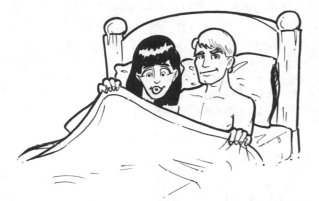

Chapter 22

Bigger Isn't Necessarily Better: Penis Enlargements

In This Chapter

➤ Accepting your penis size

➤ Consider surgical procedures only as a very last resort

➤ Making sure the risk is worth it

➤ Alternatives to surgery

When it comes to penis size, all men are not created equal. Penises come in a variety of different shapes and sizes, and while two penises might be the same size when they are flaccid, they may be very different sizes when they are fully erect. The reverse is also true. Two penises that are the same size when they are fully erect may also be quite different sizes when they are completely flaccid.

It's not fair, but we are not all created equal in the department of penis size. In some cases, the differences in penis size can vary quite a bit.

All Men Are not Created Equal

The parts of the penis are the same for all men who were born anatomically correct. The size of each part is usually what varies the most from man to man. The most obvious difference in penis size is usually detected in the length and girth of the shaft of the penis. The shaft of the penis is largely responsible for sexual arousal and pleasure for both partners during intercourse, and a study by Masters and Johnson reveals that girth of a man's penis size plays a key role in the level of sexual satisfaction for women.

The penis is composed of the base, the shaft, the corona, the glans, the frenulum, the scrotum, and the testicles. Although these are all important features, the most noticeable features to men and their partners during intercourse are the size of the shaft of the penis and the scrotum. Both are features that many men would like to enlarge and have silently sought cosmetic treatment for over the last 50 years.

Making a Big Deal out of It

Many men have been so unhappy with their condition that they have sought penis-enlargement procedures that eventually proved to be unsafe and ineffective. These procedures are illegal today but are quietly practiced in some parts of the world on unsuspecting patients. We encourage you to review the following procedures and not to let yourself become a statistic. If a surgeon offers any of the unsafe procedures listed below, report him or her immediately to your local medical board.

Penis-Lengthening Surgery

During the 1960s, penis lengthening was performed by a few surgeons who actually did increase penis size. This was achieved surgically by loosening the ligament that attaches the penis to the pubic bone, marching it forward, and then resecuring the attachment between the pubic bone and the penis. In many cases, the reattachment was not made strong enough to keep the penis in place. This made thrusting movements during intercourse an impossibilty and resulted in bleeding and tearing of the penis. In other cases, a small central nerve that plays a key role in erectile functioning was accidentally cut, leaving some men with severe erectile dysfunction or a complete inabilty to achieve or maintain an erection. Others experienced severe numbness of the penis and a drastic decline in sexual pleasure. Obviously, the lengths that were achieved in these cases were not worth the risks and loss of penile functioning that some men endured.

Silicone Injections

Silicone injections were attempted in the 1970s in Las Vegas by some surgeons. It was believed that injecting silicone into the shaft of the penis could cause permanent enlargement and increased girth. Doctors and patients alike were horrified to discover that the silicone would migrate and eventually create uneven and lumpy shafts. (Once large doses of silicone are injected into your body, they are almost impossible to remove because of the way that they bond with your internal tissues). This treatment resulted in deformity of the penis and permanent sexual inactivity. Both of these treatments and many of the surgical treatments available today can have similar results and are accompanied by the same risks of deformity, erectile dysfunction, sexual dysfunction, and permanent impotence. We suggest that you seriously consider these risks before you decide to undergo a penis-enlargement procedure.

Penis Enlargement Options

Before you decide to surgically enlarge your penis size, there is an important fact that we would like you to keep in mind: The average penis size is six inches in length. Some penises are longer and some are shorter, but most men do not have penises that are extremely long or extremely short.

Men who are extemely well endowed or less endowed are the exception, not the rule. Many surgeons already realize this fact and do not practice penis-enlargement surgeries because of the extremely high risks that accompany these procedures. Like us, they would recommend that men seek psychological counseling to learn to accept their penis size before electing to have cosmetic surgery. Consider this fact before you convince yourself that you are a candidate for any of the penis-enlargement procedures that are available today and that are listed below for you to review.

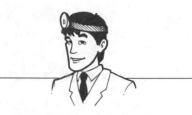

The Doctors Are In

The best treatment for a less-than-average penis size is self-acceptance. It is safe, you are completely in control of the outcome, and in many cases, it can be completely free!

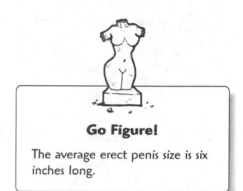

Go Figure!

The average erect penis size is six inches long.

Suspensory-Ligament Release Surgery

This surgery involves cutting or "releasing" the suspensory ligament that helps to attach the penis to the pubic bone. The suspensory ligament is responsible for holding an erection in an upright position. Without this attachment, an erect penis will stand straight out or slightly downward instead of straight up. It can give the appearance of a larger penis but does not make the penis necessarily longer. The results are permanent and can affect sexual functioning.

Pubic Liposuction

Sometimes, fat tends to engulf the base of the penis and conceals the full appearance of the penis size. Liposuction of the pubic area can remove the fat and create the appearance of a larger penis by removing the fat that prevents the entire penis from being seen. This is an optical illusion and not a surgery that can increase actual length or girth. Liposuction may need to be repeated in order to maintain full results.

Scrotum-Recession Surgery

Sometimes, the scrotum is wrapped around the shaft of the penis and it causes the shaft to look shorter than what it actually is. Scrotum recession is a surgical technique that recesses the scrotum and allows the full size and form of the shaft of the penis to be seen. Results are permanent and carry with it all of the risks of any penis-enlargement surgery: scarring, deformity, asymmetry, erectile dysfunction, and sexual dysfunction.

Cost: $3,000 or more.

Penoscrotal-Webbing Release Surgery

In other cases, the scrotum is attached to the underside of the base of the shaft of the penis in such a way that it conceals the actual size of the penis. Penoscrotal-webbing release surgery severs part of this connection and accentuates the definition between the shaft of the penis and the scrotum. It gives the appearance of a larger penis, and results are permanent.

Cost: $3,000 or more.

Dermis Fat Grafts or Fat Injections

Dermis fat grafts or fat injections involve removal of the fat from one place on your body and the reinsertion of it to the shaft of the penis. This can increase penis girth—with severe risk of deformity and all of the other complications that can accompany penis enlargement surgery.

Fat has a tendency to be absorbed by the body once it is reinserted. This can leave the penis looking lumpy and bumpy. In addition, the glans or the head of the penis cannot be made larger through dermal fat grafts or fat injections. This means that the shaft of the penis can be made larger, but the head of the penis must stay the same size. The two can end up looking very disproportionate if the surgery is a "success" and the fat is not reabsorbed by the body.

Cost: $3,000 or more.

Combination Surgery

A combination of any of these surgeries can be performed to increase the appearance of penis size. However, we do not recommend that any of these procedures be performed.

All of these surgeries are currently available and can be practiced by any medical doctor. This means that an eye surgeon can operate on your penis! This is a very scary proposition when you consider that this surgery already has potential risks for devastating complications. If you do elect to have any of these procedures performed, be sure that your surgeon is board certified in both urology and plastic surgery. This is not the type of operation to entrust to someone who does not specialize in urology or does not have an expert understanding of penis functioning.

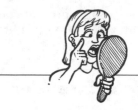

Wrinkle Ahead!

You might end up trading function for form if you choose a surgeon who is only certified by one board.

When Size Matters: Nonsurgical Treatments

If you have tried counseling and no amount of psychological assistance can help you to feel better about your penis size but you do not want to have surgery, then there are some nonsurgical options available that can help you to increase the length and girth of your penis and cause your scrotum to look larger. These are uncomfortable and time-consuming techniques that will require diligence and patience on your part. However, because they are nonsurgical techniques, they are considered to be the safest form of penis enlargement.

Before you move ahead with any of these techniques, keep in mind that they can increase the size of your penis, but gains of more than two inches are almost impossible to make, even with continued use of the following nonsurgical methods:

Penis Pumps

Penis pumps are vaccum devices or pressurized cylinders that men can place around the penis to increase length and girth. The cylinders come in different sizes and fit over and all the way down the shaft of the penis so that end of the device rests securely against the base of the penis and is usually held in place by hand. A handheld pump that is connected to the device is then used with the other free hand to create suction and enlarge or stretch the penis. This can be a pleasurable experience for most men and the suction is maintained for as long as it is tolerable.

Prolonged use of the device on a daily basis with increased periods of time (10 minutes each day for one week, 15 minutes each day the next week, etc.) can produce increased length and girth after several months. The amount of growth achieved depends on original penis size and the ability of your skin to stretch. Larger cylinders can be used as growth occurs. Results are not immediate and must be maintained by repeated treatment.

We recommend that you not exceed 20 minutes of use per day, avoid falling asleep with the device on, and consult with your doctor to see if this procedure is right for you.

Testicle Extenders or Penis Rings

Testicle extenders or penis rings can be used to stretch the scrotum skin and cause the testicles to hang in a lower position. These items are usually made of plastic, rubber, or leather. They are short strips of material that are fastened around the top of the scrotum and above the testicles. They are not placed around the shaft of the penis itself. Prolonged use of these devices can cause extension to occur and give the appearance of a larger scrotum.

These are the only two nonsurgical techniques for penis enlargement that are considered to be both safe and effective treatments. There are several versions of vacuums and testicle extenders available over the counter today. Any other over-the-counter treatments on the market today are not recommended at this time until longevity of their safety and dependabilty of their effectiveness have been established.

The Least You Need to Know

➤ The average penis length, when erect, is six inches.

➤ Seek counseling before you consider any penis lengthening or thickening operations.

➤ Make sure that any surgeon who operates on your penis is a certified urologist and plastic surgeon.

➤ An effective penis-enlargement technique that carries the least amount of risk is the penis pump method.

➤ Testicle skin can be stretched nonsurgically to give the appearance of a larger scrotum.

Part 6

Happier Skin and Hair

We can't overlook the importance of the role that skin and hair play in the field of plastic surgery. They have literally changed the face of cosmetic surgery, along with the faces of thousands of people!

Most of the procedures that are used to cosmetically improve both skin and hair are nonsurgical techniques. This is great news for those of us who do not like surgery or who faint at the sight of blood. For those who are faint of heart, the following techniques for scar revision, laser resurfacing, chemical peels, soft-tissue augmentation, hair transplants, and hair removal will yield exciting information. You'll be excited to discover all of the incredible ways that most of these nonsurgical options can improve your appearance.

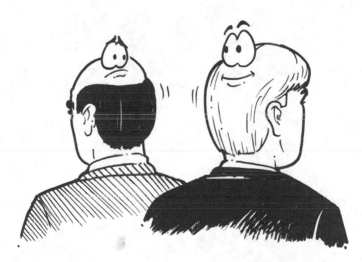

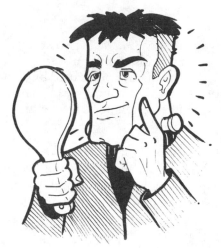

Chapter 23

Now You See It, Now You Don't: Scar Revision

In This Chapter

➤ What you need to know about scars

➤ Scar-revision techniques

➤ How to prepare for and recover from scar-revision procedures

➤ What to look for in the future of scar revision

Scars are an unpleasant fact of life. Depending on where they are located, they can be an unsightly blemish on an otherwise beautiful body part. The bad news is that almost everyone has some kind of scar. The good news is that no matter what skin type you have or how severe your scar appears to be, it can be treated, although not everyone responds well to treatment.

This chapter will help you to understand the types of physical scars, why they develop, and what exactly you can do about them. We'll tell you about every scar-revision technique available so you'll be aware of the most up-to-date procedures for improving your appearance.

Common Scars

We all know that scars are usually caused by injury or surgery, but we bet you didn't know that there are four different types of scars. The three most common scars are keloid scars, hypertrophic scars, and depressed scars. These are usually caused by surgery and are normally treated nonsurgically. The fourth most common scars are traumatic scars; they are usually the result of injury and can often be treated with surgery.

➤ **Keloid scars** are benign skin tumors that cause a thickening of external scar tissue. This is a result of a body that "overheals" itself and happens naturally among some people. Keloids do not extend beyond the scar itself and the scar raises to cause a welt-like appearance. Keloid scars are difficult to treat and they do recur.

➤ **Hypertrophic scars** are a widening of the scar tissue that causes the scar to thicken and spread outside of the scar area itself. When this happens, it usually occurs two months after some kind of surgery at the site of a previous surgical incision. They are caused by crush injury, infection, stress at the site, or too much motion at the site.

➤ **Depressed scars** form a crevice or a deepening of the skin. They can come in different shapes and sizes (like a small round depression left from a chicken pox or a long straight depression left from hair transplant surgery). Some people are predisposed to this condition.

➤ **Traumatic scars** are large or deep imperfections that can sometimes result from injury (and occasional surgery) and can be reduced through scar-revision surgery.

All types of scars can develop during any healing or recovery process and can easily be improved by the treatments discussed in the next section of this chapter. Each of these treatments can improve the color, contour, and texture of each imperfection.

Scar-Revision Treatments of Choice

There are several nonsurgical and surgical techniques for improving the appearance of scars and helping the skin to look its absolute best. We discuss the most common techniques below.

Cortisone Injections

Cortisone shots are usually the treatment of choice for most keloid scars. In this case, diluted amounts of cortison or other steroids (like Kenalog) are injected into the keloid area, and the cortisone aids in reduce or bring down the inflamed or raised scar. This treatment can help to reduce the size, shape, and thickness of the keloid.

Pressure Dressings and Bandages

Compression with bandages or other methods of applying pressure are commonly used to flatten out or reduce keloid scars. Often a tight bandage will be used in conjunction with a silicone-gel dressing to remedy the raised appearance of a keloid. Some doctors also use massage or other techniques of applied pressure to reduce its height and texture.

Collagen Injections or Other Filler Substances

Collagen injections or injections of other filler substances are frequently used to plump up the appearance of depressed scars. There are many semi-permanent substances on the market today that are available through your dermatologist's or cosmetic surgeon's office. (Be sure to read Chapter 25, "Get the Skin You Want Now! Soft-Tissue Augmentation," for a detailed description of each substance.)

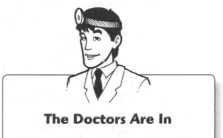

The Doctors Are In

Discuss different alternatives with your physician and choose an option that best meets your needs.

Z-plasty Technique

A Z-plasty is a surgical technique that is reserved for scars that might be limiting joint movement or where the skin is too tight. For instance, if there is a scar on the inner elbow that prevents you from stretching your arm out perfectly straight, a Z plasty may be performed to reshape and lengthen the scar to give you a wider range of motion. Z-plasties are used primarily on skin surfaces that cover joints like elbows, wrists, fingers, and toes.

W-plasty Technique

A W-plasty is a surgical technique that transforms a scar that is in a straight line into a scar that is in a zigzag or *W* shape. This was done with the hope of improved healing. Unfortunetly, it tends to look unnatural regardless of where the scar is located. This procedure is very rarely done today.

Reexcision

Reexcision is the most common treatment for revising scars. Reexcision is an operation that requires your physician to anesthetize your skin and surgically remove the entire scar. This can be a risky procedure because the scar could develop again in the same place, and there is a chance that it will be worse than the one you wanted revised. At this time, there is no accurate way for doctors to determine what the final result from a reexcision will look like. Fine scars should be left alone.

The Cost of Scar Revision

Obviously, some scars are going to be more expensive than others to treat. Tiny scars that are only slightly depressed may only need a little collagen injection that could cost well under $500 (if the scar is very, very small). Larger scars that require surgery, like reexcision, would clearly be more expensive—up to $5,000—because of the medications (numbing solution and possible antibiotic) that would be needed during and after the operation. Consider your options and discuss the cost of each with your cosmetic surgeon.

Gearing Up for Your Procedure

OK, so you've decided to do it—you're going to have a procedure or surgery performed to help improve the appearance of your scar. You don't have to be nervous, just informed! Consider the following advice before actually moving ahead with a scar-revision operation or before deciding to have your doctor revise a previous revision.

Let Mother Nature work her magic.

Sometimes the best cure is Mother Nature! She has a miraculous way of allowing your body to heal naturally, and this is sometimes a perfect way to get the best result. Let your scar heal naturally before deciding to have scar-revision surgery. It can save you time and money. And remember, when it comes to healing, Mother Nature is one of the best (and the least expensive) in the business!

Wait at least nine to twelve months before deciding on scar revision surgery.

Having scar-revision surgery before your scar has had time to heal fully increases your chances of getting a more noticeable scar, because it can impede your body's own natural healing process and can create even more scar tissue. In addition, it can create too much tension and cause the wound to heal too tightly. It takes at least nine months (really, nine months to a year) for a scar to heal. After a scar has healed completely, a doctor can accurately estimate whether or not the scar needs to be revised.

Wait until your wound or scar has completely healed before you decide to consult your physician about scar-revision surgery or any other similar procedure.

Some skin types are more prone to keloid.

Some skin types are more prone to develop keloid scars than others. And just because you may develop keloid scars on one part of your body, it does not necessarily mean that you will develop them on another part of your body or in the same place if you are having a scar-revision surgery performed. Unfortunately, there is no accurate way of diagnosing when, where, and how many times you will develop keloid scars.

Get several opinions!

Remember, scar-revision surgery (like all cosmetic procedures) is both a science and an art form. Different doctors might choose to revise the same scar in different ways. One doctor might suggest surgery while another doctor might suggest an injection. Both options could be the scientifically correct procedure, but one may be a better artistic solution and be more aesthetically pleasing to you in the long run. Get several opinions from different doctors and choose the alternative that best suits your needs.

Learn about your nonsurgical options.

There are plenty of nonsurgical options for scar revision. All types of scars usually can be improved by either compresses or injections as an alternative to surgery. Such nonsurgical treatments can change the color, contour, and texture of your scar. There are many alternatives to choose from, so be sure to read Chapter 25 on soft-tissue augmentation to learn all about your nonsurgical alternatives for scar revision.

You should consider all the risks involved in scar revision before moving ahead with this type of surgery. While there is less risk involved with nonsurgical scar-revision techniques, they are usually semi-permanent—the effects can wear off. Surgery is a more permanent solution and can have longer-lasting effects.

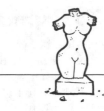

Go Figure!

Frequently, people run to their cosmetic surgeon's office as soon as they see a scar beginning to develop. Sometimes cortisone shots, pressure and silicone dressing can help. There are no guarentees.

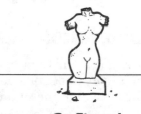

Go Figure!

Some people of Asian, African, and Caucasian descent have a risk of developing keloid scars. The cause is genetic, and while no race or skin color is immune, the formation of these scars seems to be most common among Asians.

What To Expect Afterward

Once you've had your procedure performed, you're going to want to know what to expect next. Knowledge is power, and the more you know the better you'll be able to estimate whether you received a satisfactory result from your procedure or surgery. You'll also be able to take care of yourself and plan an effective aftercare program for yourself. (Read the Chapter 28, "Taking Care of Yourself," to learn more about aftercare following a cosmetic procedure or surgery.) Here are some important facts and helpful hints.

It takes a year to see final results.

Don't be too hasty in deciding whether or not you like the final results of your scar-revision surgery. It takes one full year to see the final results. Making any decisions about how your surgery turned out before that time frame would be premature. So be patient and wait at least one full year before determining whether or not you want your physician to surgically revise your scar-revision surgery.

Some bruising is common.

Anytime an incision has been made in your skin that requires stitches, you can expect there to be some mild bruising (depending on the severity of the incision and the tension of the sutures that are used to close the incision). To help reduce bruising during and after your surgery, you might want to ask your physician about Arnica. Some health experts believe that Vitamin K, when used orally before surgery, can help to reduce bruising because it improves the clotting mechanism.

Expect some swelling.

You can anticipate some swelling after a scar-revision procedure. If your scar revision required an injection, swelling will be minimal (if at all) and dissipate quickly. However, if your scar revision required surgery, your swelling might be more acute and take several days to go away. While swelling is normal, extreme inflammation is not. If you experience extreme inflammation, see your doctor immediately.

There is a risk of infection.

As with any surgery, there is a small risk that infection will set in after your scar-revision surgery. However, if your scar revision required an injection instead of surgery, there is less risk. Keep a close eye on your incision area to make sure that signs of infections, such as extreme inflammation, tenderness, redness, and pain do not persist. If they do, call your doctor right away!

Don't wear makeup immediately after surgery.

If you're like most people, you'll want to hide any stitches or incisions with makeup or other cover-up products. Don't! Makeup and other creams or lotions (especially ones that have alcohol and perfumes) can irritate your skin and complicate your healing process. Don't wear makeup or apply any other products to the area of your face or body that has been operated on until your doctor has given you his or her approval.

Follow your doctor's instructions.

If you have chosen your doctor well, she or he has been well trained and has performed scar-revision surgeries numerous times. He or she will be very familiar with the common side effects and with any and all risks involved with your surgery. For this reason, listen closely to your doctor's instructions and follow them exactly. Make sure that when you leave the doctor's office you have an aftercare program outlined for you. That will help you achieve maximum results!

Try Aloe.

It is a common belief among many health-care professionals that topical aloe ointments and other salves or soothing solutions that contain aloe can help speed up the healing process of most incisions or wounds but there is no scientific proof that validates this claim. Vitamin E tends to cause scars that are healing to spread and becomes vascular. Once the site has healed, very small doses of topical Vitamin E are helpful.

The Doctors Are In

We recommend that you don't use Vitamin E while your scar is healing because it may cause your surgery scar to spread.

Avoid the sun for one full year.

To ensure proper healing, avoid exposing the scar you had revised to the sun for 12 months so that the area can fully regain its normal color. Exposing the area of your skin that has been surgically revised before this time could cause permanent discoloration of your skin.

After reading this chapter, you should be prepared to have any necessary scar-revision technique performed. You've probably known for quite a while what scars are problematic for you; now you are aware of how to have them fixed. There are so many ways doctors can diminish the appearance of your scars and help you regain the natural texture and complexion of your skin. And even better methods of improving the appearance of your skin are being developed.

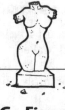

Go Figure!

Research in the field of intrauterine surgery (operating on a fetus while it is still in the womb) reveals that surgery can be performed on a fetus with no resulting scar tissue whatsoever. This gives credence to the idea that Collagen 3 (which the fetus is made up of before 3 months) may play a key role in healing a wound completely with no scar tissue. Bovine amniotic fluid (from cows) is already being used in many over-the-counter products. Breakthrough discoveries such as these suggest that with further research, experts might be able to find a way for everyone eventually to have less scar tissue after an operation ... or even a scar-less surgery!

The Least You Need to Know

➤ Don't let your scars keep you from being the most beautiful you can be.

➤ Allow scars to heal completely before considering scar revision.

➤ Consider surgical or nonsurgical options for reducing the appearance of scars.

➤ Avoid the sun for one full year after scar revision.

Chapter 24

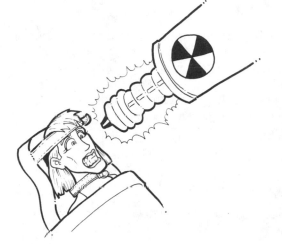

Deep Facials: Chemical Peels and Laser Resurfacing

In This Chapter

➤ What chemical peels and laser resurfacing can do for you

➤ Learning about the different techniques

➤ Preparing for a procedure by taking care of your skin

➤ What to expect after a procedure

There are wrinkles, and then there are WRINKLES! And if you're like most people, you wish you could get rid of all them, along with other effects of aging and the sun, such as poor skin tone and discoloration. If you have any of these characteristics, or acne scars, then you'll be pleased to learn that there's probably a solution for you. Over the last few decades there have been many developments in the field of dermatology and skin rejuvenation. The alternatives to rejuvenating your skin are as varied as they are common. All of the skin-rejuvenation techniques you will find in this chapter have been approved by the Food and Drug Administration (FDA) and are available in most cosmetic surgeon and dermatologist offices. Some are even available in salons.

While all of the techniques in this chapter are FDA-approved, their availability and use are subject to change depending on advancements in medicine and technology. What's here and hot today could be gone tomorrow. Any one of these techniques could be replaced with something even quicker, more effective, or with fewer known or unknown side effects. Be sure you're acquainted with all of the possible risks involved with each skin-rejuvenating procedure before you decide that any one of these procedures is for you!

Chemical Peels and Your Skin

There are a variety of facial peel substances and technologies that can be used by your dermatologist or cosmetic surgeon. They come in three different categories. There are superficial chemical peels, medium chemical peels, and deep chemical peels (or laser resurfacing). Each type of peel helps to exfoliate dead or damaged skin and gives your face a healthy-looking and more radiant glow.

The different categories of peels penetrate different levels of facial skin. The deeper the peel is, the more it will rejuvenate your skin:

➤ Superficial peels exfoliate and rejuvenate the top-most layer of your skin. They can rejuvenate your skin by making it smoother and refreshed and can have some effects on fine wrinkles and discolored skin.

➤ Medium peels penetrate below the top layer of skin to rejuvenate the medium layer of skin. They can smooth out rough skin, remove some fine wrinkles and discolored skin, and increase skin tone.

➤ Deep peels penetrate even deeper than medium peels and rejuvenate your lowest levels of skin. Deep peels require the use of either a phenol peel or laser resurfacing. They have dramatic effects on wrinkles, including the dynamic wrinkles such as the horizontal forehead creases, scowl lines between the brows, crows feet, and vertical lines around the mouth. They are also effective at removing discoloration, smoothing out rough skin, and improving skin tone. Phenol peels really are not used by most surgeons any more.

In this chapter we'll discuss the different peels in greater detail so that you'll know what kind of peel, if any, is the right one for you.

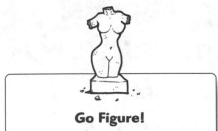

Go Figure!

What's the difference between the facial peels available over-the-counter at the local drug store and those that can only be performed by a dermatologist or cosmetic surgeon? You get quicker results that require healing time in a doctor's office and slower results that do not require a healing time from over-the-counter products. And over-the-counter procedures usually aren't as effective.

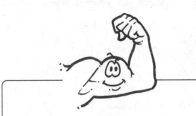

Better Definition

Dynamic wrinkles are caused by repeated movement of the facial muscles. They can appear on the forehead from raising eyebrows, between the brows from scowling, around the eyes from squinting, and around the lips from pursing them (and smoking!).

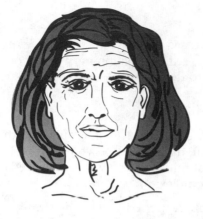

The most common dynamic wrinkles are forehead creases, crows feet, scowl lines, and vertical smile wrinkles.

The Price of Beauty

Every beauty has its price—and it's not always just financial! When considering whether to have a skin-rejuvenation technique performed, you should be aware of the financial *and* potential physical costs involved.

Although most outcomes of peels are desirable, the chances of complications do increase with the intensity or each peel or laser-resurfacing procedure. The complications can include:

➤ Discoloration. The discoloration can be in the form of darker skin or lighter skin. People with olive or dark skin are more at risk for dark discoloration, and people with light skin are at higher risk of light discoloration.

➤ Scarring. Scars are more likely to develop during medium to deep chemical peels and laser resurfacing.

➤ Cold Sores. Some people develop mild to severe cold sore outbreaks after facial peels. Be sure to take your cold sore meds prior to surgery.

➤ Milia. Tiny white bumps sometimes develop after treatment, which will eventually go away but might last several months.

You will also be more sensitive to the sun, and should plan to stay out of the sun or wear sun block after your treatment.

Be sure that you are fully aware of all risks involved and that you can afford all financial and physical costs involved. Ask your doctor about all possible side effects when considering the following procedures.

Superficial Treatments

Superficial peels, like all the peels discussed in this chapter, involve the application of a chemical to the surface of the skin to remove the top-most layers of skin in order to bring the newer, fresher layer of skin to the surface.

AHA Peels

AHA peels are made up of Alpha Hydro Glycolic acid, and out of all the peeling solutions discussed in this chapter, they are the gentlest on your skin. AHA peels are very effective at reducing the appearance of fine lines and wrinkles as well as improving the color, tone, and texture of your complexion.

These peels come in different prescription strengths, with the stronger prescriptions producing better-looking skin. Some AHA peels can cause mild skin irritation (prolonged redness and increased or decreased pigmentation), with the risk of irritation increasing the higher the strength of the peels.

These procedures take no more than 30 minutes in your dermatologist's or cosmetic surgeon's office. Patients typically have this procedure repeated once a month for a period of six months in order to achieved the desired level of success, and then they have maintenance peels every two to three months thereafter.

Particle Skin Resurfacing

Particle skin resurfacing does not require the use of a peeling solution or laser. Instead, the procedure enhances the appearance of your skin by using a highly controlled spray of fine aluminum oxide crystals that is protracted and retracted under pressure through a vacuum-like instrument. The crystals make contact with your face, buff the top layer of your skin, and then are instantly sucked back up into the vacuum.

This 30- to 40-minute procedure must be performed in your doctor's office by trained professionals. Particle skin resurfacing is highly effective in treating blackheads, whiteheads, fine lines, wrinkles, superficial age spots, and oily skin. It is recommended for all skin types, and results can be seen immediately. Anesthesia is not required.

Medium Peels

Medium peels are applied similarly to superficial peels, except the chemical penetrates the skin at a deeper level.

Medium peels can be performed with phenol with greater safety than with TCA which is better for more superficial freshening peels. These peels are generally applied without sedation because they sting only for a minute or two, and are done slowly.

They are dressed with ointment. This ointment is soothing and aids in the healing. Covering these peels with tape or dressings is generally no longer done because it makes the peel to deep and causes the pain.

Your doctor can tell the end point of the peel because it turns red as the peel is applied. This is followed by a white frost which lasts a few moments and is the signal to apply the soothing ointment.

This peel is ideal for both fine and fairly deep lines. It doesn't replace a facelift. They tend to last for years, but can be repeated every 6 weeks or so until the desired result is obtained.

TCA Skin Peels

TCA is a peeling solution that contains trichloro-acetic and comes in different strengths. TCA peels penetrate very deeply, causing the top layers of cells to dry up and peel off, and leaving you with skin that is newer, undamaged, smoother, and more evenly toned.

TCA peels, which can only be performed in your doctor's office, are enormously successful in improving dull, weathered skin, freckling, blotchy pigmentation, sun damage, fine wrinkles, and shallow acne scars. Two to three minutes of stinging or burning sensations are common side effects, so you might want to request a mild sedative from your doctor before you begin your treatment. These treatments usually take no more than 20 to 30 minutes. TCA peels have a lower safety rate than phenol as a medium peel.

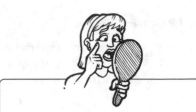

Wrinkle Ahead!

People with dark brown skin should consult with their physician about the higher risks for skin discoloration with medium chemical peels.

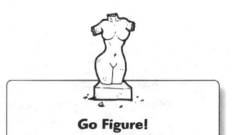

Go Figure!

Medium Phenol peels are generally safe on foreheads, eyes, nose, lips, and chin. When used on the cheeks there can be a line of demarcation.

Deep Peels

Deep peels penetrate the deepest layer of skin it is safe to penetrate, and thus have the most dramatic improvement on your skin. They are the only peel that is effective for diminishing or removing dynamic wrinkles, and they also might be effective on acne scars.

Before and after a full face deep chemical peel. Note the dramatic improvement in dynamic wrinkles.

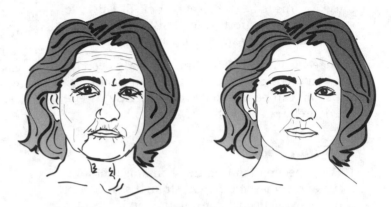

Phenol Peel

Phenol peels are deep peels that use phenol, a chemical, to penetrate deep levels of your skin. Phenol peels are conducted in your doctor's office and take anywhere from 60 to 90 minutes to perform. These can be painful, but usually only sting for a few minutes. Sedatives and anesthesia are optional.

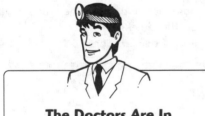

The Doctors Are In

Phenol Peels should only be performed on people with fair skin. There is a high risk of skin discoloration for people with dark or olive skin.

Phenol peels, which have been used for 30 years, have been successful in treating stubborn lines, deep wrinkles, sun damage, acne scars, uneven complexions, and other facial imperfections.

Laser Skin Resurfacing

Laser skin resurfacing involves the use of extremely short bursts of high-energy laser light to vaporize the top layers of your skin that have been weathered by age, injury, surgery, or the sun. The heat of the laser also causes the collagen under your skin to contract, which will give the exposed layer of your skin a tighter and smoother appearance.

Laser skin resurfacing has been extremely effective at diminishing the appearance of fine lines and wrinkles around the forehead, eyes, lips, and nose, as well as improving the overall tone, texture, and quality of the skin. The two most common lasers used today for laser skin resurfacing are the CO2 Laser and the Ebrium: YAG Laser, though the CO2 laser is being used less and less today.

There is currently some speculation among medical experts that the use of laser could eventually cause skin discoloration and could even cause the skin ultimately to thin instead of thicken. If this turns out to be true, laser skin resurfacing could be promoting the appearance of aging instead of preventing it.

What a selection! There are skin-rejuvenation techniques for almost every skin type. If you are considering any of the options described in this chapter, including laser resurfacing, be sure to consult with your doctor and make sure that he or she is up on the latest developments within skin rejuvenation and laser technology. It's changing all the time!

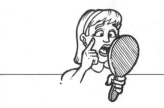

Wrinkle Ahead!

Phenol peels cause permanent whitening of the skin. If you have a lot of freckles, they will permanently remove them, as well. You can decide whether smoother skin is worth the trade-off.

Chemical Peels and Laser Resurfacing Aren't for Everyone

Unfortunately, not everyone is a candidate for chemical peels and laser-resurfacing treatments. When these procedures have been performed on people of color, such as Asians, Latinos, and African Americans, the results frequently have been unfavorable. Some common unfavorable results are

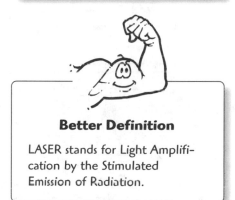

Better Definition

LASER stands for Light Amplification by the Stimulated Emission of Radiation.

hyper-pigmentation (darkening of the skin) or hypo-pigmentation (absence of skin color). For this reason, medium to deep peels are usually not recommended for people of color. If you have an olive complexion to your skin, you also might not be a good candidate for some or all of these treatments. Usually, fair-toned people with light eyes are the best candidates for peels and laser resurfacing. This is because these procedures usually result in a lighter skin color, and this effect is less noticeable on those who are already fair or pale-complected.

There is some good news, though! People who are not candidates for peels generally do not need them because they already have extra-protective melanin in their skin that acts to protect it from the signs of aging (like wrinkling). Most people of color, like Asians and dark-complected people of African and Indian (Asian) origin, do not need to be peeled.

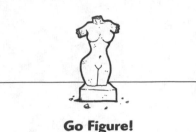

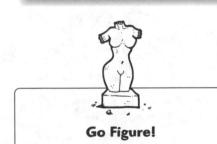

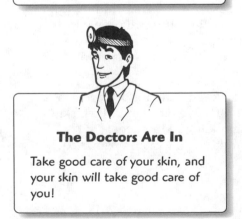

Get Ready!

So you've decided that your skin could benefit from a skin-rejuvenation procedure! Maybe you want to improve your skin tone and eliminate those tiny wrinkles that are forming around your eyes. Or maybe you want to reduce the appearance of severe wrinkling or acne scars. No matter whether you've opted for a quick and simple superficial peel or a deep-penetrating laser or chemical peel, there are things you should do to get ready for the procedure. Preparing for your skin-rejuvenation procedure is just as important as the procedure itself. How you take care of your skin before your treatment can have a direct effect on how quickly and well your skin heals.

Here are some helpful hints to assist you in taking care of yourself and to best prepare you for a speedy recovery!

Avoid sun tanning.

In order for your treatment to go smoothly and your results to be the absolute best, avoid sun tanning for several weeks before your procedure. Tanning can make it difficult for your doctor to estimate which areas of your skin need the most treatment. It can also complicate your healing process and cause discolored skin to develop. Many doctors will not perform these skin-rejuvenating procedures on anyone who has recently been in the sun or on anyone who has a sunburn.

Cleanse and moisturize daily.

Maintaining the youthful appearance of your skin requires cleansing and moisturizing your skin twice a day (once in the morning and once at night). It is recommended that you cleanse your face with a cleanser that is specifically designed for the softer, more delicate skin of your face. Moisturizing your skin after you cleanse your face is essential to maintaining the soft and smooth texture of your face. Moisturizers can also help to maintain the elasticity of your skin. Clean and moisturized skin is healthy and beautiful skin!

Consider using antiwrinkle creams.

Using Renova and other antiwrinkle creams can help to prepare your skin for your chemical peel or laser resurfacing treatment by giving you a jump start on diminishing fine lines and wrinkles. Renova is the only FDA-approved medication that can help to reduce wrinkles and decrease the effects of chronic sun exposure. Renova also has been proven effective in lightening brown spots (age spots or sun spots), reducing blotchiness, and leaving complexions clearer, smoother, and less lined. Renova can be used nightly, and after desired results have been achieved, it can be applied three to four times a week to maintain its effects. It is available only by prescription.

Drink plenty of water regularly.

In order to fight wrinkles from developing or deepening, your skin needs to stay hydrated. Drinking plenty of water (at least eight 8-ounce glasses a day) will give your skin the hydration that it needs to stay firm and supple.

Maintain a well-balanced diet.

A well-balanced diet that provides your body with proper nutrition is essential to maintaining a beautiful tone and texture to your skin. If you are not drinking enough water or eating well enough, the results (usually a dry and sallow complexion) will ultimately show on your face. A well-balanced diet and vitamin supplements can supply your body with adequate nutrition and keep your skin looking fresh and radiant!

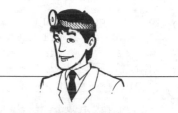

The Doctors Are In

We recommend drinking eight 8-ounce glasses of water everyday, and even more when you are exercising or involved in rigorous activity.

Remember, these are not face-lifts.

Chemical peels and laser resurfacing will help to reduce fine lines and wrinkles. They will leave your skin softer and smoother. But they are not face-lifts, and thus will not improve the appearance of sagging or drooping skin (read Chapter 5, "Turning Heads and Breaking Hearts: Face-Lifts," for information on surgical procedures to correct sagging and drooping skin). Putting these helpful hints into action will help you to get your skin into tip-top condition before your procedure. More importantly, it will help you to maintain the positive results of the skin-rejuvenating technique that you choose. Don't forget: Take good care of your skin, and your skin will take good care of you!

Now That It's Over

Once you've had your procedure, it's time to relax. If you've had a deep peel or laser resurfacing, we mean *really* relax, as you'll need to devote seven to 10 days at least recovering from the procedure. Read on and find out exactly what to do now that it's done!

Superficial Peels

Superficial peels have very little, if any, side effects. Occasionally there is mild redness, irritation, or some minute flaking of superficial skin. However, the fact that you've had a peel is usually undetectable—except that your skin will look more fresh and radiant, of course!

You should be able to resume your regular routine immediately after your procedure—you can even return to work right away. Anesthesia isn't required for this type of a peel, so there is no down time. You can drive right after you leave your doctor's office and there is little to no risk of infection or other complications after having this procedure done.

The results of superficial peels last for a few months, and the procedure will need to be repeated (on an as-needed basis) to maintain the glowing results of your superficial peel.

Medium Peels

Because medium-depth peels usually require a mild anesthetic, you will be unable to drive immediately after your peel is performed. It would be best to plan to have a friend take you to and from your doctor's office on the day of your procedure.

You will also experience severe peeling for the next three to ten days. If you have a medium peel performed, we recommend that you schedule some time off work after the procedure and follow your doctor's aftercare instructions precisely.

You will need to keep your face moisturized and avoid picking at your face or peeling the skin off. Instead, allow the peeling to happen naturally.

Possible but uncommon side effects of this procedure include infection, irregular pigmentation (discoloring or blotchiness of the skin), activation of herpes (cold sores), and scarring. This procedure can reduce the appearance of scarred and sun-damaged skin. It also creates a fresher and more youthful look. Results can last up to one year and may eventually need to be repeated.

Be sure to stay out of the sun for at least six months after your treatment to prevent blotchiness and to keep your skin looking its best!

Deep Chemical Peels and Laser Resurfacing

Because deep chemical peels and laser resurfacing penetrates the deepest level of skin possible, your facial skin will be very raw immediately following the procedure. This raw skin is extremely sensitive and very fragile. It is highly susceptible to infection and injury and must be dressed with petroleum jelly and bandaged for two to five days. Dressing and bandages will need to be changed twice a day. Frequent checkups with your doctor will also be necessary during this crucial recovery time to detect and prevent any infection (such as yeast, viral, or bacterial infection) from occurring. It is critical to your recovery and the ultimate appearance of your skin that you keep your face moisturized and bandaged for several weeks after your treatment. Otherwise, drying, cracking, scarring, and irregular pigmentation could occur.

The skin that will develop after this treatment will be newer, smoother, and tighter than before. The results of this procedure are permanent and will not need to be repeated. Avoid staying out of the sun for at least six months to a year after having a deep peel or laser resurfacing.

Intravenous sedatives are commonly used during this procedure, so be sure someone will be available to take you home from the doctor's office. You'll also want to take at least 10 days off from work.

Take a Sneak Peak

Recent developments in laser research suggest that newer lasers that are quicker and more effective in stimulating collagen-producing cells could be here sooner than we think. The development of this technology could also mean that the results of your treatment will be easier to predict and the occurrence of some side effects will be reduced. Someday, all of us could defy Mother Nature and enjoy younger-looking skin for longer than she had originally intended!

Congratulations! You are now fluent in skin rejuvenation and laser resurfacing. You are equipped with all of the necessary knowledge to make a fully informed decision about which procedure will best meet your cosmetic needs. You can review these facts any time you need to. Choose your options carefully and select wisely!

The Least You Need to Know

➤ Consider using superficial peels to remove superficial dead and damaged skin.

➤ If you have mild forms of sun damage or want to soften fine lines, medium peels might be the procedure for you.

➤ Opt for deep peels or laser resurfacing if your skin is sun-damaged or you want to soften deep lines.

➤ Make sure that you're a good candidate for peels or laser resurfacing before undergoing the procedure.

➤ Always avoid the sun for at least six months after having any kind of peel or laser resurfacing.

Chapter 25

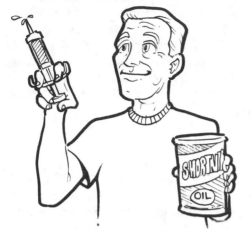

Get the Skin You Want Now! Soft-Tissue Augmentation

In This Chapter

➤ Putting an end to aging

➤ Understanding your options for reducing signs of aging

➤ Getting the scoop on the most popular soft-tissue-augmentation choices

➤ What you can expect your recovery to be like

You can't stop time, but sometimes you can slow down the effects it has on your appearance ... and without surgery! Soft-tissue-augmentation procedures remain the latest and greatest nonsurgical techniques of choice for those wanting to diminish the appearance of facial lines around their forehead, brows, eyes, mouth, and neck.

With soft-tissue augmentation, there are a variety of innovative ways to correct facial flaws such as deep worry lines in the forehead, frown lines between the brows, crow's feet around the eyes, smile lines that travel from the outside of your nostrils to the outer edges of your lips, and scars created by acne, injury, or previous facial surgeries.

Soft-tissue augmentation also can be used to plump up your cheeks if they have lost their fullness due to age or chronic illness. Botox can even lessen the appearance of what some call "chicken bands," the vertical lines in the neck that begin under the chin and travel downward, which most commonly occur in older women.

Soft-tissue augmentation is the process of injecting FDA- approved material such as collagen into the face to correct unwanted facial flaws and to restore the appearance of fuller, smoother, and more youthful-looking skin. Desired results are usually achieved through a series of injections, but also can require implantation through occasional surgery. In the next few sections we'll tell you what soft-tissue-augmentation options are available, which options are the most popular, and how to plan for your procedure, as well as what to expect afterwards. At the end, we'll let you in on what the future holds for soft-tissue augmentation.

Decisions, Decisions

There are several kinds of soft-tissue augmentation, and you might find it difficult to determine which is the best procedure for you. This is a common problem, and we'll help you overcome it by describing the procedures, indicating what procedures work best for what problems, and estimating the costs. No matter which of the procedures you end up selecting, you can be assured that all have been approved by the FDA and are both safe and effective.

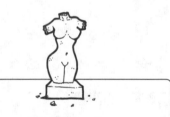

Go Figure!

As you can imagine, this is a popular technique because patients get to plump up one area of their body while simultaneously ridding themselves of a little unwanted fat from another area.

Fat Injections

Ever wish you could get rid of unwanted fat from your buttocks, thighs, hips, or stomach? And what about diminishing the appearance of deep lines in your face or neck? If you answered "yes" to both questions, then do we have a solution for you! Fat injections use your very own fat—taken from a part of your body where you would like to have it removed—to plump up deep lines in the face and neck. Fat injections leave patients with a younger-looking face and a thinner body. Who wouldn't love this minimally invasive option?

Your doctor makes a small incision prick in the skin in the area you want fat removed and extracts the fat with a syringe. The fat is then prepared for reinjection by isolating it from all other blood and residual materials. Your doctor then reinjects the fat into your skin in an area where your wrinkles are the deepest. General anesthesia is recommended but not required.

Fat injections are usually reserved only for very deep lines because it is a bulkier material than most of the other augmentation alternatives. Local anesthetic is required, and mild bruising and swelling may occur. (Not all fat that is extracted will survive the procedure, so your surgeon will have to inject more fat than what you actually need) There is a brief recovery time ranging from a few days to a couple of weeks,

and the results can last for up to eight years. Because fat is composed of natural biological cells, over time some of the cells will shrink, and some may die. It takes up to
eight weeks to determine what kind of follow-up treatments will be needed; such
treatments will most likely be necessary for more lasting results.

Estimated cost: Varies according to procedure and series of injections, but usually
$2,500 or more.

Dermis Fat Grafts

Dermis fat grafts, also called fat transplants, involve the excision of a deeper layer of
the skin, and extracting and implanting larger volumes of fat, and surgery is normally
required. Dermis fat grafts are usually taken from your body when you are having a
procedure such as a tummy tuck or a fanny tuck done. Since you are already under
anesthesia and incisions have already been made into the more fatty areas of your
body, it is a convenient time for the doctor to extract a large amount of unwanted fat
from one or more of these areas and reinject it into an area of your body (such as
your face or even your hands) that could benefit from its use. You can expect your
body to absorb some of the transplanted fat, so occasional follow-up treatments will
also be required.

Estimated cost: Varies according to operation and series of grafts, but usually $3,000
or more.

Fascia Transplants

Fascia is another natural substance that is taken
from your own or someone else's body (such as a
human-cadaver donor). During fascia transplants,
fascia is usually surgically removed from the upper
part of the leg of a cadaver and is then reinserted
into an area of your face to help diminish the appearance of deep scars or stubborn wrinkles.

Anesthesia is required for this surgical procedure
and no recovery time is usually necessary. Most
people are able to return to work and their other
daily activities in one to two weeks. Like fat grafts,
fascia transplants yield semipermanent outcomes.
Mild bruising and swelling can occur. Follow-up
sessions will be required to achieve satisfactory results.

Estimated cost: $2,500 or more per procedure.

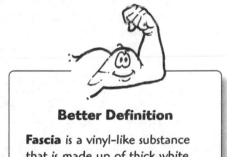

Better Definition

Fascia is a vinyl-like substance
that is made up of thick white
sheets of connective tissue that
are located in a deeper layer of
your skin around the muscles.

Fascian Injections

Fascian is an injectable form or fascia and has only become available recently. The substance is extracted from a human-cadaver donor and is then procured (rehydrated) and processed into a thick solution that is made up of solid bits and fibrous materials. This material is then injected into the severely lined or depressed areas of the face or hands.

The body naturally absorbs fascian and scar tissue usually forms around it, holding the fascian in place and preventing it from moving. As a result, it is not usually dissipated into the rest of the body. If your body does not easily digest fascian, the effects from your fascian injection can last for years and possibly even decades. However, many people see the effects dissipate between six and twelve months. Redness or swelling may occur immediately after the procedure. Follow-up treatments will be needed for long-term maintenance. It is important to note that Fascian has not been out long enough to say whether or not it should be your treatment of choice.

Estimated cost: $1,000 per procedure.

Collagen Injections

Your body is naturally made up of collagen. When the collagen in your skin starts to thin, wrinkles begin to form. The wrinkles will deepen as the collagen continues to thin.

Injections can replenish your skin with the necessary collagen to smooth fine lines and wrinkles, as well redefine the size and shape of your lips. Occasional and temporary swelling can occur, but there is no recovery time. The results of collagen injections are immediate and can last anywhere from three to six months.

Estimated cost: $350 per cc of collagen. The amount of collagen varies according to a person's needs and preferences.

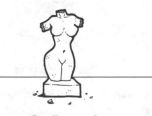

Go Figure!

Collagen is a natural product of the skin. It can be obtained from cows (bovine collagen), from human cadavers, or your own body.

Zyderm and Zyplast Implants

Zyderm and Zyplast implants are a different form of collagen injection and are the only soft-tissue-augmentation materials that contain lidocaine, a numbing solution that helps patients feel more comfort while the procedure is being performed.

Zyderm and Zyplast are both usually well tolerated by the body if you are not allergic after skin testing. They are moldable after they are injected. Some inflammation can occur immediately after the procedure but it usually dissipates quickly. No anesthesia is required and there is no recovery time. Results can be immediately detected and last from three to six months. Follow-up treatments are always required to maintain a desirable result.

Estimated cost: $350

Isolagen Injections

Isolagen is an injectable material that is made up of collagen-producing cells. It is extracted from your own body, procured and processed in a lab, and then reinjected into an area of your face that is either deeply lined or scarred. It can also be injected into your lips to give them a fuller and shapelier appearance. Two to four treatments are usually necessary to achieve desirable results. This is a relatively new treatment and although it has been approved for use, we still consider this to be an experimental treatment until it has proven its effectiveness for a greater length of time.

The effects of Isolagen injections are semipermanent and can last up to two or more years. This treatment is not recommended for patients over the age of 60, since their bodies do not contain appropriate collagen-producing cells. Some burning and stinging may occur during treatment, so anesthesia is recommended. Follow-up treatments will eventually be necessary.

Estimated cost: $500 per cc of Isolagen.

Autologen Injections

Autologen is injectible collagen that is extracted from your own body during a surgery like a face- or brow-lift, a breast reduction, or a tummy tuck. Your own collagen is removed from a fatty area of your body that is being operated on and then sent to a laboratory to be processed for reinjection. This process takes three to four weeks.

Once your collagen has been procured into autologen, the autologen is reinjected into creased and lined areas of your face to give it a smoother and more youthful appearance. Anesthesia is required and results are seen immediately. The effects of autologen injections are semipermanent and vary depending on how many treatments you have. The results of autologen can last from three months to a year and beyond. Because it has not been out for longer than 20 years, we consider Autologen (and the following description of "Dermologen") to be a new and experimental substance that is subject to change with the development of new substances in the ever-changing field of medicine.

Estimated cost: $1,000 per cc of autologen.

Dermologen Injections

Dermologen is a human-derived substance (it comes from tissue banks that have received it from tissue donors) that consists of collagen, elastin, and glycosaminoglycans. All of these substances are very helpful in plumping up wrinkled skin and giving you a more youthful appearance. Like most soft-tissue materials used to diminish the appearance of facial lines, the results can be seen immediately.

The effects of dermologen are semipermanent and can last up to one year and beyond. Some stinging and burning sensations are common side effects during the procedure, so anesthesia is recommended. You'll most likely need three treatments over a six-week period (with two weeks break in between treatments) to achieve your desired results. Follow-up sessions will also be required for long-term maintenance.

Estimated cost: $133–$200 per cc of dermologen.

Alloderm Sheets

Alloderm is another collagen-like substance that also comes from tissue banks and tissue donors. The tissue banks convert donated skin tissue into a pure, human-derived form of collagen; in other words, alloderm is a processed form of collagen that comes from someone else's body. Alloderm comes in sheets which your doctor can shape and insert under your skin to diminish wrinkles, scars, and other depressed areas of your face. Small incisions and a few stitches are required to perform this operation.

The results are seen immediately and are long lasting but not permanent. Some shrinkage has been observed. Bruising, swelling, and occasional infection can occur. This is considered a minor surgery and you may need time to recover before returning to work. No follow-up treatments are usually needed.

Estimated cost: $700 per unit of alloderm.

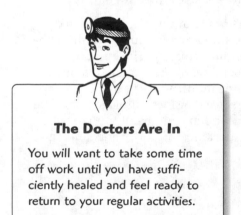

The Doctors Are In

You will want to take some time off work until you have sufficiently healed and feel ready to return to your regular activities.

Gore-Tex Grafts

Gore-Tex grafts are synthetic materials that come in solid forms (thin strips or threadlike shapes). These grafts can be surgically implanted under your skin to diminish the appearance of prominent lines or depressed scars. They can also be used to redefine your lips or increase lip size.

Small incisions and some stitches are required for the Gore-Tex grafts procedure, and anesthesia is required. You can see immediate results after your surgery and the grafts can last up to several years. Bruising, swelling, and occasional scarring or infection are often temporary side effects. In rare cases, the Gore-Tex can protrude through the skin, which would require you to have an additional surgery to correct the defect.

Botox Injections

Botox is a muscle-relaxing substance that is derived from bacterium (Botulinum Type A, to be exact). When injected into the facial muscles, botox creates temporary paralysis, relaxing the muscles and causing wrinkles to disappear.

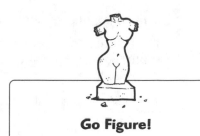

Go Figure!

Botox has been used safely and effectively for over 10 years on thousands of patients.

It is a procedure that can be done in a matter of minutes in a doctor's office with no recovery time. You will need to stay upright and avoid massaging the injected areas of your face for three hours following the procedure. Otherwise, the botox can travel to another area of your face and cause paralysis; for example, if you lay down or have a facial massage after your treatment, the botox that was injected into your forehead could travel down into your eyelids, causing them to droop or even close for several months.

It takes two to three days to see the full effect of your botox injections, and the results last from two to six months. Follow-up treatments are required for long-term maintenance.

Estimated cost: $10 per unit (the eyes average about 20 units, 20–50 for forehead).

Silicone Injections

Silicone injections have been banned by the FDA because of the complications that they cause and the risks that they pose to patients' health. Although the procedure is illegal in the United States, some doctors still provide these services. If your doctor recommends this procedure, he does not have your best interests in mind and needs to be reported to your state medical board immediately.

Estimated cost: This illegal procedure can cost you your looks and ruin your appearance. Don't do it!

The Most Popular Choices

Isn't it just amazing that there are so many easy ways to give yourself the gift of younger and smoother-looking skin? Most of these procedures are quick, and some are relatively painless. With fat injections, dermal fat grafts, fascia transplants, collagen, Zyderm, Zyplast, Isolagen, autologen, dermologen, alloderm, Gore-Tex, and botox to select from, which one should you choose?

The most popular selections are collagen and botox. Here's why:

Collagen injections have been the long-standing treatment of choice for patients who want to look younger as quickly as possible. The benefits of going with collagen injections include:

➤ They are one of the least expensive soft-tissue-augmentation procedures available.

➤ They offer a speedy remedy for most wrinkles and other depressed areas of the face.

➤ There is no recovery time.

➤ They have a semipermanent result.

You can see why collagen injections are the number one choice of many patients for improving their appearance.

The benefits of botox, the other most popular soft-tissue-smoothing procedure, include:

➤ The procedure is available at a reasonable cost.

➤ The results are semipermanent.

➤ The procedure can reduce the appearance of prominent lines and stubborn wrinkles almost immediately.

Gearing Up!

Once you've selected a soft-tissue-augmentation procedure and a doctor who you feel comfortable with (see Chapter 4, "Choosing a Doctor Who's Right for You"), you're ready to gear up for your procedure or surgery. That means learning what's in store for you! Here are six things you should keep in mind after you've made your selection.

Harvesting

No matter which soft-tissue-augmentation procedure you choose, your substance of choice will need to be "harvested" or extracted from somewhere (unless it is Gore-Tex). If your augmentation alternative is bovine or is human-derived from cadavers or tissue banks, then your doctor will probably already have your substance of choice on hand and available for your procedure. If you are choosing a soft-tissue-augmentation procedure that requires the use of your own collagen, fat, or other tissue, then an initial session will be necessary for your doctor to harvest these substances from your body. Not all doctors do this, but some do. If you choose this alternative, be sure to have some anesthesia for the sake of your own comfort during the procedure.

Patience Is a Virtue

Remember, if you are planning to use your own collagen, fat, or other tissue for your cosmetic procedure, this material will not only need to be harvested, but it will also need to be processed. In many cases, this requires the material to be sent to a lab to be properly prepared before it is reinjected into your body. This can take anywhere from two to four weeks.

Also, your desired results will probably not be achieved after just one treatment. You will most likely need several treatments in order get the results that you want. Keep these facts in mind and try to be patient.

It's Not Right for Everyone

Unfortunately, not everyone's system naturally accepts soft-tissue-augmentation material. In some cases, patients experience allergic-type reactions, get an infection, or reject the material for other reasons. It is rare that this happens, but it does occur. File this in your memory bank and talk to your doctor about all of your soft-tissue-augmentation alternatives if one of them does not seem right for you. Allergic and other unusual reactions are uncommon but not impossible.

Skin Test—No Need to Study!

During your initial consult with your doctor, he or she will probably give you a skin test. The doctor will inject a small amount of the material to be used in your procedure into your arm and ask you to come back in a few days to see how your skin reacted to the injection of soft-tissue-augmentation material. Collagen skin tests are read at 30 days repeated and reread fifteen days later.

If everything looks fine, he or she will most likely continue by giving you your first full treatment. If the injected area is red or swollen, or shows other signs of complications, then that augmentation option likely is not for you.

The Occasional Biopsy

A biopsy is a sample of tissue that is extracted from your body and then sent to a lab for examination and processing. Biopsies are rarely used for most soft-tissue-augmentation procedures. However, some augmentation alternatives that involve using your own tissue, like Isolagen injections, do require a biopsy.

Give Yourself Enough Time

Many soft-tissue-augmentation procedures are considered "lunchtime procedures"—in other words, they are performed quickly and easily in a doctor's office, and the patient is ready for everyday activities almost immediately. However, there are some soft-tissue-augmentation alternatives that require surgery. You should plan to spend at least two hours in the doctor's office for these procedures and give yourself enough time to heal before returning to work. Autologen, alloderm, fascia, fat grafts, and Gore-Tex implants all involve surgical procedures and will require some recovery time (usually no more than a few days to a few weeks).

If you keep these things in mind, your trip to your doctor's office should go very smoothly.

On the Road to Recovery

Once you've had your procedure performed, it's time to shift gears and find out what you can expect during your recovery period. We'll tell you about some of the most common things people experience ... but don't usually tell their friends. Remember, you have a right to know everything!

Minor Burning and Stinging

The injected areas of your face (or hands) may burn or sting immediately after your procedure. This is a common reaction and it dissipates quickly. You can reduce burning and stinging during and after your procedure by requesting that your doctor use an anesthesia or numbing cream before and during surgery or ice afterward.

Minor Bruising and Swelling

In some cases, minor bruising and swelling might occur right after your procedure. This is a common reaction and happens most often after surgical augmentation procedures are done. If you experience minor bruising or swelling, use ice to reduce the swelling and avoid massaging the injected areas to prevent further inflammation or bruising from occurring. Both side effects should begin to go away in a day or two.

An Exaggerated Appearance

Most doctors realize that your body will eventually absorb some or all of the material that is inserted under your skin. For this reason, many doctors overfill an injected area with a substance of the patient's choice. This way, your body will initially absorb the excess substance and you will be left with the appearance that both you and your doctor intended you to have. It will also keep the depressed area of your face fuller longer. Unfortunately, this means that you may have an exaggerated appearance for the first day or so until the swelling decreases and your body begins to absorb the injected material.

Temporary Numbness

Many of your augmentation alternatives require anesthesia or a numbing cream to help you feel more comfortable while your procedure is being performed. Most numbing agents used during these kinds of procedures do not last longer than an hour. If you elected to have some form of anesthesia during your procedure, expect to experience some temporary numbness after you leave your doctor's office.

Speedy Recovery

Remember, there is good news! One of the best things about nonsurgical soft-tissue-augmentation procedures is that there is little to no recovery time needed. If your procedure did not involve surgery, you can anticipate a speedy recovery!

Redness or Small Bumps

Occasionally, some people experience redness or small bumps in the areas that have been injected with their substance of choice. This is usually a temporary reaction and is nothing to worry about. However, if the redness and small bumps persist, notify your doctor immediately. He or she may want to prescribe a medication that will help reduce these side effects.

Watch for Infection

A skin test or a biopsy can usually reduce your chances of developing an infection or other complication after your procedure. Sometimes, unforeseen infections or other complications can occur. Taking antibiotics that are prescribed by your doctor before your procedure can help. If you experience severe and persistent swelling, redness, pain, or any other unusual side effects, call your doctor immediately.

Follow-Up Treatments

All soft-tissue-augmentation procedures yield semipermanent to permanent results; however, permanent results are less common than semipermanent results. Keep this in mind and plan to schedule follow-up treatments in order to achieve and maintain the appearance that you want.

Now you're completely prepared to move forward with the information and confidence you need to select a soft-tissue-augmentation procedure that is right for you.

Flash Forward!

Now let's flash forward and take a peek at the future of this exciting field! The focus of much anti-aging research (including cosmetic surgery research) will center on rejuvenation. It will concentrate on ways that medicine and technology can help to restore the skin's natural youthful appearance and maintain its smooth and full texture.

Substances like Isolagen and new technology like non-ablative laser resurfacing, which could possibly stimulate the growth of collagen in the skin, will probably become more widely researched and marketed. If these products and others can restore some of the collagen to people's skin, all of us may be able to look younger longer! Also, keep an eye out for antioxidants and hormone replacement therapy to play a key role in your rejuvenation process.

The Least You Need to Know

➤ Soft-tissue-augmentation substances can come from cadavers, cows, and your own body.

➤ Ask your doctor about having an initial skin test to see how your skin will react.

➤ Most procedures have semipermanent results, so follow-up treatments will probably be necessary.

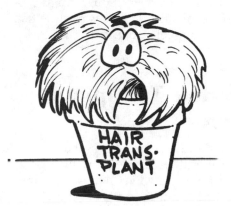

Chapter 26

Hair Transplants and Removal

In This Chapter

➤ The facts about hair and hair loss

➤ Hair-transplant surgeries and the risks involved

➤ How to prepare for and recover from hair-transplant surgery

➤ What you can do if you have excess facial or body hair

Have you noticed that your hair has lost some of its rich color and youthful luster? Is it less full, or is it receding? Do we dare even suggest that it could possibly, maybe, in bright light and up close, even be balding? Nah. Well, OK. Maybe.

Or maybe you have a full head of hair, but you would love to have smooth underarms and legs, or a bikini line that's free of unwanted hair?

If you fit either one of these descriptions, then you'll want to read this chapter to find out what options—surgical and nonsurgical—are available for you.

Learn the Hairy Facts About Hair Loss

Thinning hair and noticeable hair loss is a widespread problem. Anyone may begin to experience thinning of their hair or hair loss from the age of 17 on up.

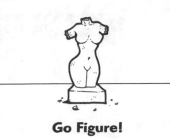

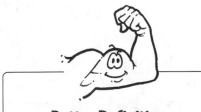

Even though women experience thinning or baldness, only men have traditionally been thought of as candidates for hair-transplant surgery. This is because hair loss in men is easier to predict than hair loss in women.

Common Hair-Transplant Procedures

From 1966 until today, hair-transplant surgery has been a common surgical technique for reducing signs of balding. The technique involves removing hair from an area on the back of the head and moving it to the crown of the head. The area on the back of the head where the hair is taken from is called a "donor site." Donor sites make up the horseshoe pattern of hair that is located right below the crown of your head and almost stretches from the back of one ear to the other. Only a narrow strip of hair is extracted from this area, so that removal of the hair will be as undetectable as possible after the surgery. It is important to note that although the following surgeries are available today in some cities, that the development of new medication that is mentioned later in this chapter is quickly replacing the prevalence and need for hair transplantation surgery.

Hair-transplant surgery is irreversible and, in some cases, it can actually speed up the natural process of male pattern baldness or cause other types of hair loss. So think twice before you have this procedure done, and make sure that it is right for you!

There are several ways to transplant hair, but only a few of the techniques offer what we consider to be acceptable results. Make sure that before you undergo any hair-transplant technique you find out from your doctor exactly what he or she plans to do, and always get a second opinion. Remember, the procedure is irreversible, and in many cases the results of a bad surgery can look far worse than what your head looked like to begin with!

Minigrafts

Minigrafts are small round areas of skin (about the size of a pencil eraser) that contain four to nine hairs that are removed from the patient's donor sites at the back of the head. These extractions are usually made with an instrument that looks a lot like a hole puncher. Before these extractions are made, very small incisions are made in the crown area of the scalp and held open with instruments that look a lot like nails to designate where the transplants will go. After the extractions are taken from the back of the head, they are immediately placed into the incisions that have been made in the crown area of the scalp. They are quickly and evenly plugged into the marked areas.

This procedure is less commonly used among many hair-transplant surgeons today. The disadvantage of this procedure, as with all transplant procedures, is that no one can really tell for sure how much hair you will lose over the course of your lifetime. So, if you get minigrafts today, you could lose all the hair on top of your head over the next several years and be left with nothing but minigrafts. You would most likely be unhappy with the "plugged look." It would be obvious to you and to others that you have had hair-transplant surgery.

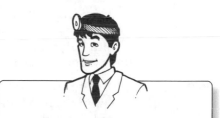

Wrinkle Ahead!

People with dark-colored curly hair usually get better results from hair-transplant surgery than someone with lighter-colored hair. Those with blond-colored hair and fair skin have a more difficult time naturally camouflaging this surgery. Dark hair does well, however, dark curly hair does best.

Micrografts

Micrografts are even smaller than minigrafts. They are small round areas of skin that contain three or less hairs and are extracted from the back of the head and reinserted into the crown area of the scalp, just like minigrafts. This hair-transplant technique is also very popular among cosmetic surgeons and is widely practiced today.

Micrografting involves the same disadvantages as minigrafting. Consider the risks, and then decide whether or not hair transplant surgery is for you!

The Doctors Are In

As a rule, a surgical hair line cannot imitate youth. It must follow lines of early recession to look as natural as possible.

273

Pattern of hair placement in hair transplantation with micrografts. You cannot restore your hairline to the point it was when you were a juvenile, because it will look like a wig.

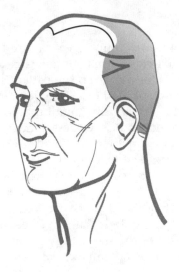

Follicular Units

Out of all the hair-transplantation procedures currently available, one seems to stand alone in its ability to produce the appearance of a fuller head of hair that looks natural instead of plugged. This procedure was developed in Sweden in the 1980s. It is the best procedure and the most undetectable.

Follicular units differ from micrografts and minigrafts in the way that they are extracted and reinserted into the head of a patient. Follicular units are units of one to two strands of hair. These units have a minimal amount of skin around them, so when they are reinserted into the scalp, the patient is not left with the appearance of plugs. It looks more like his natural hair has been grafted in rather than round pieces of skin with hair on them. In addition, the way the follicular units are redistributed into the patient's scalp also differs from most minigraft and microgated surgeries.

When we were born, Mother Nature gave most of us hairlines that began with rows of one-hair units. As Mother Nature intended, the hair in back of our hairlines grew thicker and was usually the thickest on the crown of our heads when we were younger. This thicker hair was naturally made up of one to two hair units. The follicular-unit technique redistributes similar hair units in the crown of the head, with smaller units in the front and gradually larger hair units in the back of the crown area. This gives the patient the appearance of a naturally fuller head of hair. As with all hair-transplant procedures, the same risks are involved with this type of surgical technique.

These are the surgical techniques available today in the field of hair-transplantation surgery. It's important to keep in mind, though, that these techniques are not always the most effective. Medication and future medications seem to be replacing the need for hair transplant surgery. The field of medicine and its technology are always changing. It's a well-known fact among many medical professionals that frequently more than 50 percent of medical technologies become outdated or obsolete within five years.

Hair Ye, Hair Ye!

Now that you know what the risks of hair-transplant surgery are and what kind of results you can expect from each one, you'll be pleased to hear that there are nonsurgical procedures available that have proven to be effective in some cases.

Rogaine

In many cases, Rogaine (the brand name for the topical solution Minoxidil and a registered trademark of Pharmacia & Upjohn, Inc.) has been proven to slow down the balding process in some men. It appears that it can thicken existing hair and even cause some regrowth of hair in the back area of the crown of the scalp. In order to get these results, the Rogaine solution must be applied twice daily (usually once in the morning and again in the evening) to the balding areas. Rogaine to date has not proven to cause hair regrowth on the front areas of the scalp or on areas of the scalp that are already completely bald. Rogaine is available over the counter in 2 to 5 percent solutions. It may take six to twelve months before you see any results, and this topical solution may work even better when it is used with Propecia, an oral medication. You need to continue taking Rogaine if you want to maintain your hair regrowth.

Propecia

Propecia is an oral medication (also known as Finistride, which is manufactured by Merck) that prevents testosterone from being converted in the body into dihydrotestosterone (DHT). DHT is what causes male pattern baldness in both men and women. It appears that taking one milligram of Propecia a day seems to lower the DHT levels in both the blood and the scalp, resulting in less hair loss. Studies show that the majority of men who took Propecia for one year either kept their hair or grew more hair and future hair loss was prevented. The younger you start the more effective it is.

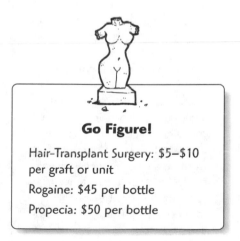

Go Figure!

Hair-Transplant Surgery: $5–$10 per graft or unit

Rogaine: $45 per bottle

Propecia: $50 per bottle

Regrowth is lost when the medication is stopped and not everyone experiences the same results with this medication. Propecia has been available since 1998 by prescription for men only.

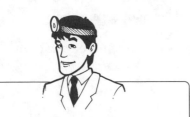

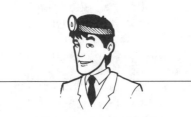

As you can see, there are a number of surgical and nonsurgical solutions that can give you the appearance of a fuller and thicker head of hair. All solutions come at a price and most require a series of treatments or some kind of maintenance. Consider these facts and select a hair-replacement therapy that fits your need as well as your budget.

Hairy Up and Get Ready!

There's absolutely no doubt that preparing thoroughly for your hair-transplantation operation will help you get a better result. Believe it or not, the most important thing to prepare before your surgery isn't your scalp, it's your mind! Preparing yourself with the right facts and the most important questions is essential to getting a great result.

Before you seriously consider having any hair-transplantation procedure, consider the following tips!

Don't expect to gain back all the hair you've lost.

Most of us are born with more than 100,000 hairs on the top of our heads. Those of us who are lucky may even have twice that. When most of us lose our hair due to male pattern baldness, we can lose up to seven-eighths of our natural hair. That leaves us and our doctors with only an eighth of our original hair to work with when it comes to hair-transplant surgery. If you've lost most of your hair and you intend to have hair-transplant surgery, be realistic. You can expect the procedure to give you the appearance of more hair, but you can't expect it to bring back all of the hair that you've already lost.

How to know who your doctor should be.

Photos can help you to understand what a doctor considers to be good work. Demonstration patients can be set up to show the best results of that office. This is usually someone who was a good candidate for the surgery. First, you need to know if you are a good candidate for the surgery, for example, if you have fairly dark coarse hair without too much loss. Next is to go to someone who did what you consider a good job from your friends and acquaintances. Remember most hair work has to be combed and blown dry to look good. Those done entirely of follicular transplants and one or two roots at a time turn out the best. Anything less than this will be a compromise and will be felt or seen when it is most important. Only follicular transplants will look good wet in the shower or pool.

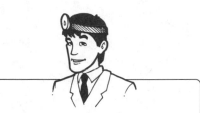

The Doctors Are In

A surgeon is only as good as his results. Be sure that the doctor you choose has given his other patients a natural-looking hair-line and the appearance of a fuller head of hair. You'll in-crease your chances of achieving the same result.

Ask your doctor how much hair is lost during an average surgery.

Since hair can only live outside of the body for a limited amount of time before it dies, some hairs are lost during this procedure. Not every transplant will in fact be able to be trans-planted. This is common during hair-restoration surgeries. Ask your doctor how many transplants he loses during an average surgery. Keep his answer in mind and look for a surgeon who loses the fewest transplants during his operations.

Choose a doctor who specializes in hair-transplant surgery.

Many surgeons can take a weekend course and become certified to perform hair-transplant surgeries. Some doctors don't even have to take courses in order to perform the surgery—they can simply watch an instructional video and then begin perform-ing the operation on their patients. Be sure to ask your cosmetic surgeon how many hair-transplant surgeries he or she has actually performed. Ask if he does the surgery completely himself or if he uses technicians to do a lot of the work. Don't allow your-self to be rushed or pressured by a doctor into making a decision on the day of your initial consultation. Your results will be permanent and rely largely on the skills of your surgeon. Also, keep in mind that medication is causing many hair surgeons and clinics to close their doors.

Avoid aspirin.

Ask your hair-transplant surgeon what medications to avoid prior to surgery. Many medications, including aspirin, can thin your blood and cause complications, such as profuse bleeding and difficulty in wound suturing, during your surgery. Listen to your doctor and discontinue any and all medications that might complicate your surgery.

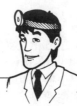

The Doctors Are In

You will most likely need several hair-transplant surgeries. Hair follicle transplants must be taken root by root from a strip of scalp hair. It is hard to place more than 1,000 roots. This is a slow and tedious process and usually makes it impossible for someone to receive the number of hair transplants that they want in just one operation. You will probably need to plan and to pay for several operations. Stopping after just one hair-transplant surgery might not give you adequate hair coverage. Keep this in mind, and schedule your surgery only when several operations are going to be within your budget.

Reduce activities and sports that might cause damage to your scalp.

It's important to protect your donor sites so that they will be in good condition and available for transplanting. Keep this in mind and limit all physical activities such as contact sports that might cause injury to your scalp or donor sites. It will help your procedure to go much more quickly and easily.

Cut your hair short.

If you are a man going for hair-transplant surgery, it might help the surgery to progress more quickly if you cut your hair short. This will make it easier for your doctor to make the necessary extractions and reinsertions into your scalp. You might also want to leave the back of your hair long enough to camouflage the area of your scalp where the extractions will be made. You will be able to comb this hair over the hair that is missing so that people will be less likely to tell that you are recovering from hair-transplant surgery.

Buy a hat or cap.

Your head will be bandaged and will need to be protected from being accidentally bumped while the swelling in your scalp decreases. Wearing a loose-fitting hat or cap can help to protect your head from any injury. It will also help to conceal the fact that you've had hair-transplant surgery. Wear the hat for cosmetic reasons as long as you need to.

Wash your hair the night before surgery.

It's important that your hair is clean before you go into surgery. Although your doctor will make sure that the conditions for your surgery are sterile, you can help speed up the surgical process by making sure that you've shampooed your hair the night before your operation. This will also save you time on the day of your procedure. In addition, be sure to avoid any activities that will cause you to perspire (like exercising) right before your operation.

All of these tips will help you to achieve maximum results from your surgery and ensure a safe and speedy recovery. Prepare yourself for success by following all of these cosmetic tips. You'll be glad you did!

Avoid a Hair-Raising Experience!

Any kind of surgery to the head is going to be a serious operation, so you'll want to take every precaution to make sure that your recovery is as safe as possible and doesn't turn out to be a hair-raising experience. Otherwise, you could end up losing some of your hair transplants! Since you'll want to keep all of the hair that you already have, follow these helpful hints while you are recovering.

Plan to take three to five days off work.

You will need to take a few days off from work to recover from your hair-transplant surgery. Your head will be swollen and bandaged for the first couple of days after your procedure, and you'll be unable to work or return to your regular daily activities. Schedule at least three full days off from work to recover from minor hair-transplant surgery (a few hundred grafts) and up to five full days off from work (or more) to recover from major hair-transplant surgery (several hundred grafts or any kind of scalp reduction).

Rest for the first 24 to 48 hours.

Your head will be sore in the places where incisions have been made in your scalp. Many patients report having the greatest discomfort in the back of the head where the extractions have been taken from, or in the area where the scalp has been reduced. This area is usually swollen and tender because of tension from the sutures that are required to close the wounds. To reduce pain and swelling, be sure to rest for the first 24 to 48 hours after your surgery.

Keep your head elevated.

During the first 24 to 48 hours after your surgery, lie flat in bed with your head propped up by pillows. Keep your head elevated above the trunk of your body so that blood does not rush to your head and increase swelling. Also, avoid all other lying or sitting postures that would place your head in a position where blood would rush to your head. These postures can slow down your healing time and complicate your recovery process. Sit and rise slowly from all lying and seated positions in order to maintain your balance.

Use cold compresses.

Keep the crown and the back of your head continuously iced with cold compresses. This will help to reduce the swelling and speed up your healing process. It is common for many people to experience a rise in body temperature after they have had surgery. Cold compresses will help to regulate your body temperature and keep you as cool and as comfortable as possible while you recover.

Take all prescribed medications.

Many people begin to feel better right after their hair-transplant surgery. Sometimes people start to feel so good that they begin to believe they do not need to take the medication that their doctors have given them to prevent infection from occurring after their surgery. No matter how good you start to feel after your surgery, don't fool yourself into thinking that you don't need to take your medication. In order to keep feeling good and heal as quickly as possible, continue to take all medication prescribed by your cosmetic surgeon until he has told you that you can stop.

Avoid getting your hair wet.

After your surgery your transplants must have time to heal too, until they have permanently connected to your scalp. You will want to avoid getting your hair wet, or your grafts may slip out of place and leave an open wound. You will also want to avoid getting your hair wet in order to reduce the risk of infection. Avoid shampooing your hair or getting it wet in any other way (like swimming) for the first few days after surgery or until your doctor has given you his approval.

Avoid strenuous activities for one to two weeks.

Avoid strenuous activities such as working out and contact sports for one to two weeks after your surgery. This should give your new transplants time to bond permanently with your scalp without running the risk of damage to the follicles or injury to the stitched areas of the scalp. You'll find that your recovery period will go much more smoothly!

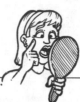

Wrinkle Ahead!

Avoid severe changes in altitude for the first 24 to 48 hours after your surgery. During this time, your transplants will not have had sufficient time to permanently bond to your scalp. Severe changes in altitude (like traveling by plane or driving up into the mountains) can create a change in air pressure. This change in air pressure can cause your unsecured transplants to pop right out of your head! Also, any turbulence during a fight could cause uncontrollable bleeding. If your cosmetic surgeon is in another city, state, or country, plan to stay in town during your recovery period. Be sure to postpone all travel plans for the first seven to fourteen days while you are recovering.

Stay calm.

Most people who have hair-transplant surgery expect to have more hair after their procedure than less hair. Some are surprised to learn that frequently they lose more hair after their surgery. It is common for other hair follicles surrounding your transplants to react to surgery by going into shock. When follicles go into shock, hair loss results. If this happens to you, stay calm. The hair loss is usually temporary and in most cases begins to grow back in a few months after surgery.

Be patient.

Most people anticipate being able to see the results from their surgery almost immediately. In other words, they wake up and expect to have a full head of hair right after their procedure. Realistically, it will take several months for your new transplants to begin to grow hair that you can comb. Keep this in mind and be patient while your hair goes through its natural rejuvenation process. You will be able to feel your new hair before you are able to actually see it.

These are the essentials to recovering as quickly and as safely as possible. In addition, if you follow these tips, you will be mentally and emotionally prepared to deal with any and all effects of your surgery. Most of all, these helpful hints will assist you in improving the overall appearance of your hair.

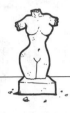

Go Figure!

A recent laboratory study has revealed some evidence that hair from other people's heads may be able to be transplanted onto your own head in the very near future.

Breakthroughs in the field of cloning suggests that you may someday be able to clone your own hair in order to grow an unlimited supply of hair for future transplanting. In addition, today's research and technology also supports the idea that dermal sheath cells (which are necessary for hair growth) could someday be cultured in laboratories and then injected into your scalp to stimulate hair growth. One or all of these theories could end up making the procedures discussed in this chapter obsolete!

Hair Today, Gone Tomorrow

Believe it or not, almost our entire bodies are covered with hair, and it grows in places on our bodies that most of us find unappealing in one way or another. For women, it grows between the eyes; along the jawline, upper lip, neck, and arms; and on the underarms, back, stomach, and legs. It grows in these places on men's bodies, too, but it is hair on the back, back of the neck, and on the shoulders that most men find unappealing and want to have removed. Unwanted hair can prevent women from wearing high-cut bathing suits, shorts, short sleeves, and skirts, while it can cause some men to be reluctant to wear tank tops and muscle shirts in the summer, or to go shirtless at the beach or pool.

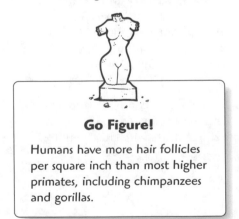

Go Figure!

Humans have more hair follicles per square inch than most higher primates, including chimpanzees and gorillas.

In the past, hair removal has required plucking, shaving, waxing, chemical depilatories, and electrolysis. Plucking, shaving, and waxing are only temporary remedies for unwanted hair, and chemical depilatories (lotions that cause your hair to fall out) and electrolysis can be painful. Electrolysis is especially painful because it calls for a needle to be inserted into your skin so that an electric current can pass through it and eventually destroy the root of your hair follicle. This prevents your new hair from growing in. Risks during electrolysis include electric shock, infection, pitting, and scarring.

Laser hair removal is the quickest and easiest way to permanently remove large areas of unwanted hair with minimal risks involved.

Going, Going, Gone!

There are several hair-removal lasers available today. However, the most up-to-date procedure for hair removal is the Light Sheer Diode Laser. This laser produces a beam of highly concentrated light that is absorbed by the pigment of your hair follicles. The laser pulses for a brief moment, then, in an instant, the pigment is vaporized and the follicles are either damaged so that regrowth is impeded or they are completely destroyed. Best of all, this particular procedure is performed in your dermatologist's or cosmetic surgeon's office with a special contact-cooling hand piece that can protect and cool the top layer of your skin before, during, and after each vaporizing pulse of the laser. Treatment time varies according to the size of the area of your body that you would like to have hair removed. Most sessions take 45 to 90 minutes. Follow-up treatments may be necessary to achieve more permanent results and most laser treatments are not effective on blond, gray, or light-colored hair.

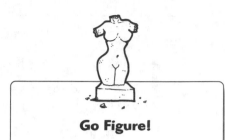

Go Figure!

The field of laser surgery is rapidly changing, and new light wave instruments might replace laser soon!

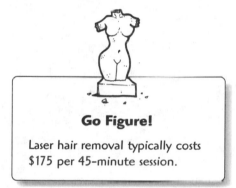

Go Figure!

Laser hair removal typically costs $175 per 45-minute session.

After your procedure you can expect to go back to work or return to your regular daily activities immediately. In some cases, redness, swelling, and small raised bumps are common. These side effects are easily treated with anti-inflammatory creams and cold compresses in your doctor's office right after your treatment. They usually dissipate within a matter of minutes. Be sure to avoid the sun after your treatment, too, otherwise discoloration of your skin could result.

The Least You Need to Know

➤ Know the risks involved in hair-transplant surgery.

➤ Understand that no amount of hair transplants can give you back the hair you've lost.

➤ Ask to meet with your doctor's patients and practice the "comb test."

➤ Laser hair removal is the quickest and easiest way to permanently remove large areas of unwanted hair with minimal risks involved.

Part 7
Let the Healing Begin

No book about cosmetic surgery would ever be complete without a section on healing. Now that you have prepared for your operation and had your surgery performed, the most important part of your cosmetic process begins—your recovery period! This is the most critical part of your entire cosmetic-improvement process, because how you heal will determine how you will ultimately look and how long your looks will last. Your appearance will rely heavily on how you take care of yourself after your operation. In order to achieve and maintain the results of your cosmetic surgery or procedure, follow the simple postoperative tips in the following chapters. Here's to a speedy and uncomplicated recuperation!

Chapter 27

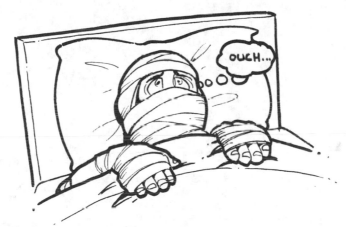

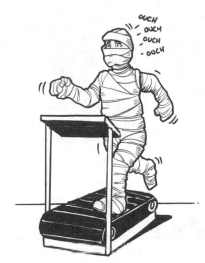

Fast-Track Healing

You've heard the facts and fiction about surgery. Now, it's time to learn the truth about healing. Everyone heals in different ways and at different speeds. But no matter who you are, there are some simple things you can learn to help you heal as quickly as your body will allow you to. Get prepared to put the myths about healing behind you and read on to discover the facts about the fast track to healing.

When you have surgery, all statistics are suspended. There is no longer a half-percent chance for a complication; if you have one, it will be 100 percent.

To most doctors, an acceptable risk of complication during or after a surgery is considered to be that one person in 10,000 people will probably experience some complication. But even risks of less than one in 10,000 are still risks, no matter how small. Neither you nor your doctor wants to take more than a one in 10,000 risk with your chances of healing.

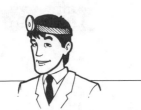

The Doctors Are In

The risks you take before, during, and after your surgery will determine how quickly you heal. The life you've lived up to the time of your surgery will affect you.

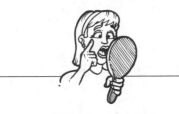

Wrinkle Ahead!

Always follow pre- and post-procedure instructions! Confessing to a mistake, such as sun tanning immediately after a deep chemical peel or running two weeks after a calf implantation procedure, doesn't mean that your doctor will be able to fix the ensuing negative results.

No matter what is done, the doctor is not working on stainless steel, he is working on your flesh that will either heal well or heal poorly. The flesh may naturally heal and leave a scar if you are genetically predisposed to scarring (this is commonly seen in noses that heal in an unsightly way). If you know the risks that are involved and the chances of experiencing complications, you can plan ahead and feel secure about your decision to have surgery.

You Pay Your Money and Take Your Chances

You can tell if you tend to scar easily (with white scars, pigmented scars, and depressed scars) by taking a close look at your hands. Because hands are injured—nicked, cut, scraped, etc.—often, they are a good place to look to determine how you heal and how you scar. Some hands are all marked up, and if there is pigment or darkening at these sites, it's not a good sign for your healing abilities after cosmetic surgery. Similarly, some people heal with white scars, which indicates that they are likely to have visible white scars from any cosmetic surgery they have performed. White scars can be tattooed the same color as your skin or be covered with makeup. But makeup is not a permanent solution. Most people who scar easily already know they do because of previous scarring from previous injuries or incisions.

Where We Heal Well, Where We Heal Poorly

As you've learned by now, everyone heals differently. Your genetic makeup has a lot to do with how you heal, but it also depends on how well you take care of yourself before and after your surgery. But did you know that different parts of your body heal differently, too? Read on for some interesting facts about how different parts of your body heal:

➤ **Extremities:** Long bones—arms, legs, the center of the chest, and the shoulder—heal poorly. If you do not heal well in these areas, your doctor will use extreme caution during surgery or might even refer you to someone else who has more experience in this area. Furthermore, scar revision is typically unsuccessful in these areas.

➤ **The mouth:** Jaws and the lip near the vermillion, the red part of the lip, can heal poorly due to the continual motion of eating and talking in this area. For wounds to heal properly in this area, they must be held still.

➤ **Reinjuring wounds:** Operating on areas that have been previously wounded is risky because it is impossible for the cosmetic surgeon to know how the wound will reheal.

➤ **Lips, eyelids, noses, nipples, and genitals:** These areas generally do not keloid. (As always, though, there are exceptions.) Location is not a dispensation of immunity, but the odds are in your favor. Plastic surgeons count on these areas to heal well with minimal scarring, which is why they make their incisions in these areas if they are able to.

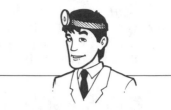

The Doctors Are In

Any risk, no matter how small, is still a risk during surgery. Ask your doctor what risks you are taking during surgery and what the odds are that a complication might actually happen to you. Any surgery that involves risks greater than 1 in 10,000 are not for you. Remember, a risk is a risk is a risk!

Don't Gamble with Your Appearance—It's the Only One You've Got!

So if you can tell by taking a close look at your hands or the color of your skin that your wounds heal poorly, or if you happen to know that you scar easily in certain areas of your body, don't expect to have cosmetic surgery and not end up with a scar or two.

Yet, it isn't wrong to trade a scar for a change, and as we've pointed out above and elsewhere in this book (see Chapter 23, "Now You See It, Now You Don't: Scar Revision"), some scars can be flattened or hidden over time by using pressure, massage, or collagen injections. White scars can be tattooed to match your skin color, and silicone coverings seem to quiet down some scars.

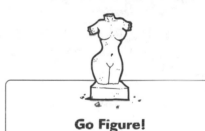

Go Figure!

Just as it is the case that long bones and fingers must be held still in order to heal properly, it is also true of skin. Problem areas that tend to scar do better if they are immobilized with tape. Placing a splint across the suture line takes the pressure off of the suture line and decreases the chances of scaring. You might have to leave it in place for two to three weeks.

So if you are planning to have surgery, make sure you think ahead to how you will heal. Remember what areas heal well and which areas have a tendency to scar in most people. The areas of your body that may be at risk for scarring are your extremities (arms and legs), the center of your chest, the area around your mouth, areas of your body that have been previously wounded in an accident. That doesn't leave many body parts left. That's why we have a little saying in the cosmetic business: You pay your money, and you take your chances!

It's the Environment

So let's say that based on the discussion above, you've determined that you're at low risk for scarring or healing poorly after your cosmetic surgery. Good for you! Does this mean you are ready to plunge in, confident that there's good chance that you'll have a speedy recovery with no scars to speak of? Not yet! There are external and internal factors that could affect how well you heal after your cosmetic surgery, which we'll discuss in this section.

Who Heals Well?

People who heal well typically have some or all of the following attributes:

➤ They tend not to gain and lose weight.

➤ They tend to have high-protein diets and take vitamins.

➤ They are not and have never been smokers.

➤ They do not have sun-damaged skin.

➤ They drink minimal to no alcohol and are happy and accepting of this.

Even if you don't have these attributes now, you can "clean up" for surgery by adopting these healthy practices now and it will still help. Cleaning up will only take a month or two. But if you go back to your old ways after your procedure, the results might not last as long.

Sun-Free and Healthy

The sun has a cumulative effect. It begins very early. The skin looks good for a period of time, and then suddenly seems to change. It thickens and wrinkles and somehow is not attached to its underlying structure. It re-wrinkles and doesn't hold a lift or peel as well as differently damaged skin.

Chronic Illness and Poor Nutrition

It's fair to say that people who have been or who are protein-deprived or chronically ill do not do well during surgery and usually do not heal well. Before being politically correct was an issue, poor protoplasm was referred to as an issue. Furthermore, if you didn't have good nutrition as a child or if you have a family history of chronic illness or are presently sickly, this could affect how well you heal. You can increase your chances of healing well by starting and maintaining a healthy diet and working with your doctor to prepare yourself for surgery. It is easier to prepare for surgery and to heal in a matter of weeks, than to do nothing to prepare and take months to heal.

Hormones and Skin

Hormone-deprived skin does not heal well, and we find that women who take estrogen look better and hold their surgery better than women without estrogen. Hormones thicken the skin and prevent wrinkles from deepening.

If You're Over 45 ...

Chronological age is not necessarily a factor in how well you heal, but physiological age is. Some people think that calorie deprivation may extend life, vitamins and antioxidants might contribute to the efficiency of metabolism, and stem-cell washing might repair signs of aging (but is so new that its uses and effects are not fully understood yet), and somatotropin (injected growth hormone) might be an effective anti-aging method. These are totally uncharted waters. We feel comfortable reporting that those on somatotropin and the other items mentioned seem to bruise less and heal faster than others, but the jury is still out.

It's not too late to start down the road to better health, and thus make yourself a better candidate for healing properly after cosmetic surgery. Make an appointment with your doctor and talk to him or her about what you can do to increase your chances of a healthy and speedy recovery!

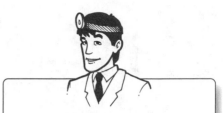

The Doctors Are In

Dr. Semel recommends that his female patients use a phytoestrogen cream, which seems to be effective for maintaining healthy skin. It has the added benefit of delivering estrogen where it is needed. It is a natural hormone that is derived from plants.

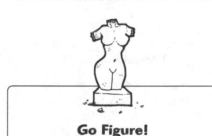

Go Figure!

The direction that current research is taking (with anti-oxidants and hormone replacement) may improve the quality and span of peoples lives.

Some People Get All the Breaks

There are people who lie to themselves and break all the rules, and seem to get away with it. If you want to maintain your health and your appearance, though, you cannot always break the rules and expect it not to catch up with you. So, although some people have the genetics that can tolerate the effects of negative behaviors such as drinking and smoking better than others, we don't recommend that you practice any

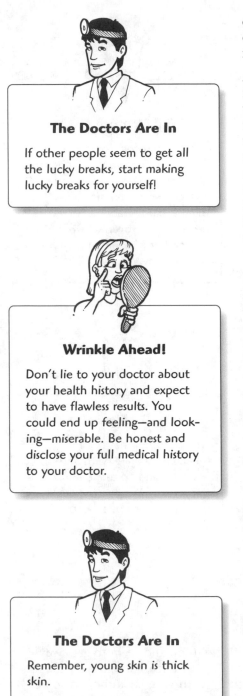

The Doctors Are In

If other people seem to get all the lucky breaks, start making lucky breaks for yourself!

Wrinkle Ahead!

Don't lie to your doctor about your health history and expect to have flawless results. You could end up feeling—and look-ing—miserable. Be honest and disclose your full medical history to your doctor.

The Doctors Are In

Remember, young skin is thick skin.

of these behaviors, particularly if you have a bleeding disorder, heart trouble, glaucoma, or other eye ail-ments.

Avoid flying by the seat of your pants or walking away from surgery with a devil-may-care attitude. People who seem to get away with these behaviors are more the subjects of urban legends than real people. People who have surgery and fly to the Caribbean for vaca-tion the next day, or those who take their nasal casts off (after nose surgery) for parties, generally have to have their surgery redone. As we have all probably learned by now, there are few exceptions to the rules in life, and the same is true when it comes to taking care of yourself after cosmetic surgery.

When It Comes to Your Health, You're the Expert!

You are the expert about your health. Only you know your full medical history, and most diagnoses are based on the patient's medical history. Your doctor will only know what you tell him or her. While we might sometimes wish otherwise, surgeons are not mind readers, and there are only a limited number of tests and screenings that are routinely performed. So be sure to disclose your full medical history to your doctor before having any cosmetic procedure done.

Ways You Can Create Your Own Breaks

No matter what your genetic predisposition is, you can become one of the lucky people who heals flaw-lessly by creating some lucky breaks for yourself. We recognize that sometimes lucky breaks aren't created by chance; they're created by a lot of preparation. Here are some tips to help you create some lucky breaks for yourself!

➤ **Limit your caloric intake.** Start your diet and see where it goes. Eat reasonably, not by fad.

➤ **Moderation in all things, especially sugar!** People with high sugar diets usually tend to age more quickly than those who don't, so for that reason alone it's a good idea to avoid eating a lot of sugar. At the same time, our brain runs on sugar, so you need some. Our advice: Practice moderation.

➤ **Sleep!** Get the rest you need so you won't be sleep-deprived before your surgery. You need to be well rested so your body can heal after your surgery.

➤ **Check out your hormones.** Ask your doctor to run tests to find out what your hormone levels are. Hormones levels have an effect on your energy as well as your ability to heal.

➤ **Treat depression.** Depression may have a slowing effect on healing. If you take medication to control depression, don't stop taking it for surgery unless instructed otherwise by your doctor. But be sure to tell your doctor what medications you are on, because complications may arise if anesthesia is necessary.

➤ **Avoid (more) sun damage.** Even if you have already done some damage to your skin by exposing it to the sun's harmful rays, there is no sense in compounding the damage.

➤ **Use Vitamin A.** Vitamin A, in the form of Retinol or sometimes retinyl palmitate, can have a profound effect on helping skin revive itself and should be part of your daily beauty regime.

Here's to Healthy Healing

Now that you know the risks involved in cosmetic surgery and what you can do to increase your chances of a speedy and healthy recovery, it's up to you to start preparing yourself—it's never too early to start. Remember, your doctor and Lady Luck can only do so much to improve your looks—the rest is up to you!

The Least You Need to Know

➤ Mentally prepare yourself for scarring after your surgery, even if the scars are difficult to detect.

➤ Don't take chances with your health after your cosmetic surgery.

➤ Increase your chances of healing faster by maintaining a healthy diet and following your doctor's instructions.

➤ Rest is the best medicine after any kind of surgery.

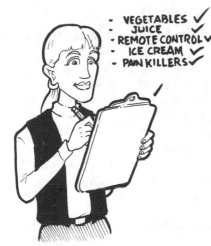

- VEGETABLES ✓
- JUICE ✓
- REMOTE CONTROL ✓
- ICE CREAM ✓
- PAIN KILLERS ✓

Chapter 28

Taking Care of Yourself

In This Chapter

➤ Your role in the recovery process

➤ Battling your inner perfectionist

➤ Maintaining a healthy diet and relaxed lifestyle

➤ Taking good care of yourself long after your surgery

Although the recovery process for any surgery is dependent on your overall health and how well you have taken care of yourself throughout your lifetime, the care you give yourself in the weeks and months following your surgery can have a big impact on your healing. And even though you can't do anything about how you lived your life before, in this chapter we'll show you what you can do now to take control over the healing process and thus do everything you can to ensure a safe and healthy recovery.

The First Seven Days After Surgery

Your first week of recovery is the most critical period of your recuperation because it is when you are at the highest risk for infection, rejection of an implant, loosening of stitches, or other complications. What happens during the first week of your recovery determines how you will heal.

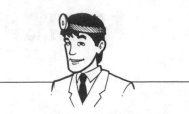

Don't Let Your Inner Perfectionist Interfere with Your Recovery

The first week after cosmetic surgery is usually the most difficult period to endure on a psychological level because of the bleeding, bruising, swelling, pain, and temporary disfigurement that most people experience. A high number of people who seek cosmetic surgery tend to be perfectionists, and living with the postoperative discomforts, even though they are temporary, can be very unnerving and disturbing.

Most people want to see immediate results and have a low tolerance level for their own healing process, especially if their body tends to heal slowly. After all, people get cosmetic surgery because they want to look better, and they usually want to look better immediately! But it's important to try to be patient and to get plenty of rest. Allowing yourself to get upset over something that you cannot control produces needless anxiety and stress. These are two anti-healing agents. A relaxed mind and a relaxed body are the required ingredients for your body to heal at its optimum speed.

Sit Back and Avoid the Mirror

Focus on relaxing and avoid looking in the mirror unless you sense that you are experiencing some type of complication. Constantly looking in the mirror when you have just come out of surgery can be a depressing and anxiety-producing experience. Allow yourself to look in the mirror or at your surgery sites only a few times a day to check for proper healing (a decrease in swelling, bruising, and pain). Otherwise, stay away from the mirror and engage in a quiet and relaxing activity like reading a book or watching television.

➤ Don't look in the mirror unless you have a sense of humor.

➤ Maintain a liquid diet for the first few days (no alcohol).

➤ Drink plenty of protein powder.

➤ Take your antibiotics.

➤ Don't over-medicate.

➤ Take your antibiotics.

The First Few Weeks After Surgery

With most major surgeries, you will continue to experience some pain and discomfort in the first few weeks after surgery. At the same time, you will begin to get restless and will want to start living your active lifestyle again. This is a crucial period in your recovery, because your body is still very fragile and there is still a risk of tearing incisions, and dislodging implants.

Maintain a Proper Diet

If you are like most people, this is the time when you will be the most tempted to turn to food for comfort or practice other unhealthy vices like smoking or drinking alcohol to cope with the discomfort and boredom.

It is important to recognize that the pain that you will naturally experience after any kind of surgery can be considered a psychological stress factor and that you will most likely be tempted to deal with this stressor as you would any other stressor in your life. This can be problematic if the only ways you tend to deal with stress are through methods that would be counterproductive to your recovery, such as overeating, smoking, drinking, or engaging in recreational drug use. Plan to use other ways of coping. (Medication and ice can also help you to manage your pain.)

Maintain a low- to moderate-calorie diet that is low in salt (to avoid swelling) and remove all of the unhealthy vices from your home that you usually use to cope with stress.

Confide in Others

Be sure to utilize a counselor and your close friends for emotional support during the first few weeks of recovery. Confide in the person you have chosen to stay with you during your recuperation if you are tempted to respond to the stress of recovery with vices that would be counterproductive to your healing. You'll find that this will help you feel and look better more quickly.

The First Few Months After Surgery

In the first few months following surgery you will probably begin to look and feel better. But just because you look well doesn't mean that you have fully recovered! You can go back to your daily activities that do not cause severe pressure or stress to your surgery sites (avoid strenuous exercise and lifting that will pull your sutures if you have them). You can maintain your daily routine but do not over exert yourself. As we've said before, a complete recovery often takes up to a full year or more for many people. It can take this long for your results to stop morphing and the reconstruction or implantation that was created during your operation frequently needs anywhere from six months to a year to become what feels like a natural and normal part of your body.

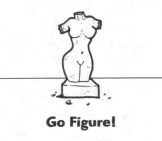

Go Figure!

Wounds are usually 89 percent healed three weeks after surgery and 98 percent healed three months after surgery (if you heal well).

Don't Become Complacent

This is the period during which people are most likely to become complacent about taking care of themselves—they figure that because they look good, they must be fully healed and can engage in any activity they want. Wrong! Don't talk yourself into believing that just because you look great, you can stop practicing self-care. Get plenty of rest and don't overdo it by jumping right back into a very busy or physically demanded schedule. It will be a long time before your body has made a complete adjustment to its new alterations, and until then we encourage you to put as little stress and as few demands on your body as possible.

Six Months After Surgery

Once your results have had time to stabilize, it is up to you to maintain those results. As we've mentioned before, your cosmetic results can leave as quickly as they came if you do not take care of them with proper rest, nutrition, hydration, sun avoidance, exercise, and care. Many people believe that once they have had their surgery that their results will maintain themselves or that they can always have the surgery repeated if they are uninterested in taking care of their new appearance.

If you don't have the motivation to maintain your results and believe that your surgery can be easily repeated later on, remember that you may not heal as well the next time if you do not take care of your body now. Keep this in mind and maintain your cosmetic results by taking excellent care of your body for six months and beyond your surgery date. Your results and the need for repeat surgeries will depend on it!

The Least You Need to Know

➤ You are at the highest risk for complications during the first week of your recovery.

➤ Don't convince yourself that you are fully recovered after a few weeks.

➤ Avoid jumping right back into a busy or physically demanding job right after surgery, especially the first 10 to 12 days.

➤ Maintain your surgical results as long as possible, because there's no guarantee that your next procedure will go as smoothly.

Index

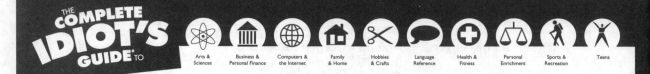